CANCER, CURRY & ME

SUVEKCHYA GHIMIRE

Book Cover Design and Illustration: Ignacio Andres Paul
Photography: Perry Graham

First Printing, 2020

ISBN 978-1-8381527-0-3 (paperback)
ISBN 978-1-8381527-2-7 (hardcover)
ISBN 978-1-8381527-1-0 (ebook)

Health Life Spice
20 Kingsgate House
2-8 Kingsgate Place
London
NW6 4TA
United Kingdom

First Edition

10 9 8 7 6 5 4 3 2 1

To *Mambaba*

Mr. Dilli Raj Uprety,

Who always thought I was a great storyteller
and knew I would write someday.

He was right.

CONTENTS

ACKNOWLEDGMENT

They say when you are faced with adversity, the true nature of those who care (or don't) can be felt and seen. During my cancer journey, I was overwhelmed with the love and messages that came my way. If I were to thank them all individually, this entire book would be covered with the names of those who helped me in life and those who were involved in helping me make my dream a reality.

Though I am grateful to each and every person who has been along this path with me, I would especially like to extend my appreciation to the people mentioned in the coming paragraphs.

To some of the most fierce women in my life, Ma, Mimi, Bri Di, Sujala Di and Bune, who passed on (and share) the "courage gene". You gave me the extra strength I needed to face cancer with all your support and good wishes.

To Ba and Aama, whose example taught me that struggle is a part of life and that those who don't give up always come out victorious.

To Baba, who has not only taught me everything I know but also has the willingness to learn from me and everyone around him - young or old. May I be more like you, strong in the belief that we are all children learning each day and with each experience.

To Mamu, whose capacity for help care has set a different standard of motherhood for me. Without you I would not be anything and without your love I would have not have the courage to face this. Thank you for being who you are. It is what has made me who I am today.

To Raj, who held my hair back when I threw up and later helped me shave it off. You put your life on hold to attend all my appointments and to be with me when I needed you most. You are my strength, my source of happiness, my energy, and my world.

The underdogs of the process who were so instrumental in bringing my book to life. Simoné Streck and team, thank you for giving my book some dazzle.

Then there are the relatives and friends who are so much more than "just" family. The love you gave me grew into courage and from that courage came healing. Thank you for healing me.

INTRODUCTION

DAWNING

> *"It was the best of times, it was the worst of times, it was the age of wisdom, it was the age of foolishness, it was the epoch of belief, it was the epoch of incredulity, it was the season of light, it was the season of darkness, it was the spring of hope, it was the winter of despair, we (I) had everything before us (me), we (I) had nothing before us (me)..."*
>
> —*Charles Dickens,*
> *A Tale of Two Cities*

How could I have known that my cancer journey was no different from a revolution? A personal upheaval that would leave its mark in some unexpected ways. Throughout my own pilgrimage, there were moments where I thought the world was falling apart, followed by moments where I felt rejuvenated and ecstatic to be alive.

The pain was so extremely unbearable that I wanted to die after every chemotherapy session. Yet, right before the next round, I had the urge to live and to do great things. This bittersweet tango became my "new normal" for a while.

In these pages, I share my cancer journey and how my life changed throughout the experience. I delve into what it taught me, and how my perspective on life has metamorphosed into something completely new. Every pilgrimage teaches us something; and in sharing mine, I hope anyone reading this book can understand cancer better.

This isn't about focusing only on the hard parts or dwelling on the negative. The fact is: there's nothing "easy" about it - any "cancervivor" can tell you that. It's a long and tough road but there is something so remarkable in it, every step of the way. In braving this path, I was given the opportunity to change my outlook on the way I experience my life, myself, my loved ones. I hope that others can find some hope in this and see a similar opportunity as they embark on their own unique journey.

I am trying to raise awareness, spread the message, and share my personal experience.

> *This book is for the brave warriors who have battled cancer and won.*
>
> *It's for those who are in the midst of their fight.*
>
> *It's for families, friends, colleagues, strangers.*
>
> *It's for everyone connected by the same thread but in different ways.*

This book is in no way intended to offend anyone's condition or situation. It is purely based on my own experience and my personal take on experiencing cancer, chemotherapy, radiation and the tremendous baggage it comes with. This is a memoir of my personal journey, and like any experiences, no two are the same.

I have divided the book into three parts: my cancer journey, some of the recipes and spices that helped me on the road to recovery, and what my experience meant to me.

Born and raised in Nepal - and now married to an Indian - I found myself craving the all-too-familiar tingle on my tongue during chemotherapy. I needed my tastebuds to feel alive. Zesty, spicy, aromatic food - heady with aromatics - that's what I wanted. It didn't matter that this was often the very reason I couldn't quell my gag reflex. I desperately needed something to overcome the new, unwelcome companion that piggybacked on my other chemotherapy side-effects: the constant taste of soap in my mouth, among many others. I didn't see that one coming.

My father is a fourth generation Nepali born in Myanmar. His side of the family has no small amount of Burmese influence in their cooking. As a result, my palette has been attuned to bold flavours from a young age. Something as robust as *Ngapi* (made from fermented fish and prawns) is no match for my tingling taste buds.

The recipes I share in this book are traditional Nepali/ Indian, from the sub-continent and beyond, passed down through generations.

The spices, herbs and recipes, are not a replacement for any treatment; rather an add-on to the recovery process. These spices are associated with Ayurveda. They are all-natural but if you're concerned about any of the herbs and spices, I'd suggest consulting a nurse or doctor.

After all, we do need a little bit of spice in our food (and life). Flavour is worth living for.

BEGINNING THE BATTLE

I began my cancer journey as a 32-year-old woman. I was in the prime of my life and the diagnosis came without warning. I was the first person in my family to be diagnosed with the disease. It made no sense. Not to me, not to anyone.

The year 2016 started off with everything feeling right. My husband and I needed to make some changes, and so our departure from New-Delhi, India was definite. Three years of working and living in a foreign city had taken its toll on our bodies and relationship. I was going to finally say goodbye to my stressful and demanding job, the noise, the traffic, and the pollution. We were waving a not-so-fond farewell to the constant need for anti-allergens and the general work-life stress that plagued us daily.

I was also going back to study and get another degree, which I had always wanted. The year had only just begun and it seemed like it was going to be the best year ever. It was a year of new beginnings in the UK.

My mother used to say, *"Dherai na hasa, runu parcha."* The literal translation of this phrase is, "Don't laugh too much, you will have to cry." It's a turn of phrase warning against being over-excited about something, lest it be balanced by a negative. In my perfect Yang, I was about to be faced by my Yin.

A few months into our new lives, it hit me - hit us - like a speeding train. The diagnosis I never dreamed I would face in a million years. It just wasn't on my radar.

As most people do, I hit Google hard, trying to find out everything I could about "my type of cancer". Breast cancer was my new nemesis; an enemy I could not yet understand. I had to do some learning first. I collected books, articles, case studies, research, and anything else I could find to try and understand my condition. After all the reading, I came to the conclusion that there are no proven facts of how and when this illness strikes. Cancer can happen to anyone.

Of course, this was something my doctors had already told me. One opinion was not convincing enough for me at that time. I had to get 2nd, 3rd, and 4th opinions. Since it was so new to me, I needed to know more. I had only heard of others who had been diagnosed via the grapevine. I never really knew anyone who had been through this battle personally.

It was pretty clear that I needed more than clinical diagnoses and medical journals to read. The personal element was missing - the "realness". I dove into any of the more real stories I could find, using social media to look for people who were in the same situation as me. Reading was a safe space; I was not ready, mentally or physically, to attend face-to-face support groups. With some time on my hands and with a somewhat patchy internet connection in my London flat, I found some great blogs and forums where I might discover the answers to a few sensitive questions like: "What can I do about my nails falling off?" or "How do I stop a non-stop stream of vomit?"

There are so many side effects that aren't discussed by doctors and nurses. Similarly, there are so many side effects that you just don't remember to ask about them when you're in the middle of yet another chemo session. Breakouts, painful eyeballs, extremely dry eyes, or any number of bizarre reactions to God-knows-what at any given moment, these are the things you deal with that nobody ever really talks about.

I met so many amazing people out there on the Internet. I learned so much more than I could have with my nose in a medical journal. But, I felt there was still something missing. I felt I needed something a little more specific to me and my heritage. I was looking for women I had more in common with that shared my experience. Though I tried to search for any information about South Asian, Indian, or Nepali women and breast cancer, very little was available. All I could find was clinical research and scientific surveys.

I was unable to find blogs of anyone desi (anyone born and raised or with family ties from the South Asian region) who went through something similar. I'm not sure whether this is because of the stigma attached to cancer or because of a cultural distaste for exposing personal vulnerabilities to the public. Maybe it's because there aren't that many young desi girls who have had breast cancer. Either way, it was a struggle that made me feel just a little more alone than I already did.

Sometimes, you just need a connection that binds your experiences - whether good or bad - to your roots. This was one of those times.

My Food, My Life

I am not sure where my passion for food comes from.

I love to eat. Could that be it?

My love for food goes beyond just travelling to a new country for new eating experiences. I take pleasure in looking into the different ingredients involved in making a dish. I want to know the secrets behind "a pinch of this" and a "dash of that". I'm in it for the entire cooking process. I want to see, taste, and feel the magic that happens behind the scenes - not simply the final result on the plate.

More specifically, after cancer, I was drawn to the ayurvedic herbs and spices I heard my grandmother and mother talking about while I was growing up. I wanted to learn more about the healing and restorative properties of the homemade dishes passed down from one generation to the next.

This was my opportunity to dig deep; to unearth more about my own food culture and history. The knowledge I've acquired on my journey goes far beyond the kitchen, far beyond the home. It's all so incredibly exciting!

How wonderful - and terrifying - to learn that at one time spices were expensive and traded illegally. Wars were started because of the spice trade. The East India Company was formed by British merchants to outthrow the trading monopoly of the Spanish and Portugues in India. It's no wonder that certain spices were so rare and so expensive. It's also not surprising that some still are. Who knew that Yarsha-gumba, more commonly known as Caterpillar fungus, is a parasitic mushroom that per kilogram is more expensive than gold? Commonly thought to have been used for its viagra-like properties, it is super potent for the immune system too. Incidentally, when my paternal grandfather was ill, this fantastic fungus gave him strength and helped him cope during kidney dialysis.

In the 17th Century, cinnamon was a prized possession. As one of the most expensive spices in the world, along with cardamom and saffron, it was only used by the wealthy as a status symbol. At the time, these spices and others were classed as luxury goods. Today, the accessibility of spices makes them affordable to a larger population, which works in our favour, because we can all enjoy the flavour and health benefits they impart.

Ever noticed the recent trend of turmeric lattes and golden milk around the US, UK, and Europe? I fussed about it and rejected it when my mom made me some at home every night while I was growing up. Now, I pay almost half my salary for a single cup. Turmeric (or curcumin) is my favourite spice. I talk about it a lot in detail later on.

My life revolves around food, though it's not my job in any way. I am not a nutritionist, just someone who appreciates good food - healthy, tasty food. It's not surprising that when I had cancer, I related everything to food. I was upset that I couldn't eat cheese during chemotherapy, and even more upset that the smell of eggs and meat made me want to take someone's eyeballs out. My favourite Jamaican curry became an unwelcome stranger. I developed a strong love-hate relationship with sushi - I craved it and hated that I either was not allowed to have (raw) fish or that the smell and sight made me run for the hills.

No one was more surprised than me when I made the decision to give it all up and to become a (mostly) plant-based, wholefood consumer. Cooking during my treatment made me realise how beautiful life is, and I began to appreciate food even more. I compared everything to food.

My love for food goes beyond the recipe chapters here, the titles of which are all names of Nepali dishes that I associated with the various experiences I dealt with during my year-long treatment process. The first chapter is called *Karela ko achaar (Bitter melon)*. This acerbic South Asian vegetable is cultivated during the warm or hot season and often made into an *achaar* to be consumed as a condiment. I was diagnosed in the summer of 2016, June. I draw parallels between the strong taste of the vegetable and the extreme emotional turmoil I faced when I was first diagnosed - bitterness personified.

I hope you can see and understand the relationship between this and my sense of humour; of trying to take things with a pinch of salt.

After all, life is too short to not laugh, or not to live a little.

And for me, life = food.

CANCER

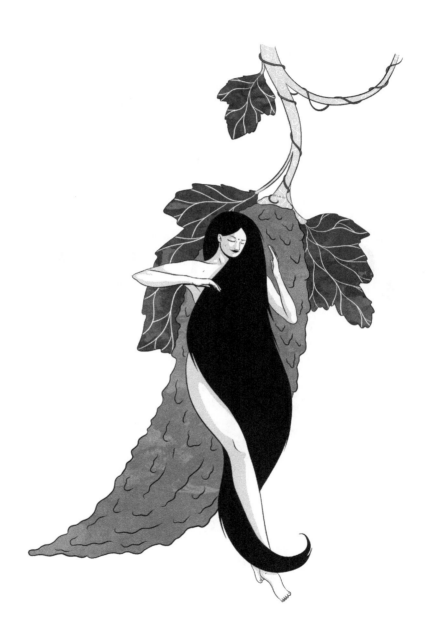

CHAPTER 1

Karela ko Achaar

A BITTER TRUTH

Karela - also known as bitter gourd or Momordica charantia - is an extremely bitter vegetable, commonly found in South Asia. Karela has many health benefits when consumed as juice or made into a saute or achaar (a Nepali style marinated salad, or relish, or pickle eaten as a condiment). This vegetable, certainly an acquired taste, is often soaked in salt water to remove its acrid taste and then cooked. Even after squeezing the soaked vegetables, it still has a strong taste that lingers in the mouth. Karela ko Achaar is a condiment made by adding a lot of tangy flavours to a bitter karela.

Just like the vegetable, discovering that I had cancer was the most bitter moment of my life. Although I internalised and came to terms with the fact over time (and I did take my time), three years on, the bitterness still remains.

Let's talk about the reality of the situation.

Why is it important to "get real"?

It's important to understand why I'm writing a book about cancer; my memoir, my experience.

With cancer on the rise, perhaps it would help to have a different outlook - a different perspective - on this new, overwhelming, and unpleasant phenomenon. To me, it's just that: a phenomenon. It's not simply a disease. There's more to it than that.

We need to hear more stories about recovery and survival. Perhaps this will help dilute the negative stigma cancer has developed - opinions and beliefs that stem from a lack of understanding and fear.

According to Wikipedia (a source so many people rely on), a disease is "a disorder of structure or function in a human, animal, or plant, especially one that produces specific symptoms or that affects a specific location and is not simply a direct result of physical injury." Cancer does not always produce symptoms, at least not in the early stages. It just doesn't fit that definition to a tee. My discovery of my cancer was just by fluke. I was at my healthiest: good stamina, decent diet, and a healthy lifestyle.

Cancer isn't something that happens only to our grandparents or uncles and aunts, or the aging population anymore. Contrary to what people used to believe, it has absolutely no age barrier. Cancer does not discriminate. With the number of cancer diagnoses on the rise, we have to find a way to deal with this condition.

There can be a lot of resentment during cancer, towards cancer. "Fuck you, Cancer," is a curse many people are all too familar with. They paint the condition as a villain - personifying it as the ultimate Bad Guy. Though it may come as a surprise, I always had a different vibe. I thought of it as a "messenger". My body was telling me that something was not right. It was forcing me to listen.

We might be able to listen to this messenger at the right moment. We might not get that all-important notification in time. Either way, it's crucial to remember that cancer isn't a disease on its own. It's a collection of cells that have mutated because of 'something.' Something important. Something we must pay attention to.

It is very likely that cell mutation happens in everyone's body. Fortunately for most, the body's immune system is able to fight it off. It doesn't let the mutation progress any further. Some of us, however, might not have the ability to fight these cell mutations. That's when simple cell replication becomes cancer.

No one has been able to find the cause of cancer. It's a medical mystery that researchers are still working on. Only the symptoms are treated. Surgery gets rid of the malignant mutated or enlarged tissues, while chemotherapy is the "cell killer". It gets pumped into the body, hoping that any cancer cells floating around will get zapped. Unfortunately, it kills both the good and bad cells - probably the ugly ones too. Localised radiotherapy basically does chemotherapy's job but only around one area.

A woman who's been a smoker her whole life might never get cancer, whereas someone who has never smoked might be a victim of lung cancer. A yogi might get cancer and so might an athlete. My family has absolutely no history of cancer. I don't know anyone (maybe with the exception of my distant relatives) who have had cancer on my dad or my mum's side.

When I was diagnosed, I often asked myself, "Why me? What did I do wrong?" I spent a lot of my time trying to figure out what made me more susceptible than anyone else. I never got answers to any of these questions because there are none.

I often thought the blame lay with me because I was not active enough, or because I did not mediate enough, or because I used to eat meat, or occasionally drink. I'm the kind of person that needs answers. I need to understand. That's just part of my inquisitive nature. Even as a child, I always needed an explanation or an answer.

I know why you get a headache if you don't drink enough water or why you feel like you're falling as you drift off to sleep. After cancer, I was left with many unanswered questions. There were no 'real' reasons for anything. There was no explanation. At some point, I realised I needed to stop asking.

Despite there being so many mysteries, I did learn that genetics play a huge role in the development of cancer. If you are diagnosed, the chances of your offspring having cancer down the line are much higher. Another weird part of the conundrum. If there's no cancer in your family, you can still get it. If there's cancer in your family, the likelihood is higher. This doesn't mean cancer is a certainty. As I said before, when it comes to this condition, nothing is certain.

Following my diagnosis, my maternal family all went for a check-up. I had to also get my genome tested (genetic test to see if cancer is in the genes) and, thankfully, the results were negative. My case was a rare and independent one.

After an hour of crying at the doctor's office, and occasionally still after that, I was rather practical about cancer. I was rational. I started to read and made myself aware of breast cancer, the treatments to follow, and what I was in for. I read blogs belonging to people who were in a similar situation to mine. I also took advantage of the facilities provided for cancer patients through the hospital and various charities.

Through a family friend, I found an amazing oncologist in India, who has had a great track record of treating many patients. I consulted him for a second opinion as I went along. I had a fantastic medical team at the hospital; doctors, nurses, and other patients I met who have become wonderful support. Many of them have given me great advice - either because they have gone through the same thing or because they are medical professionals. Regardless of all the help I received and continue to receive, there were some things *I* needed to help *myself* understand. I needed to find my own way forward.

If it wasn't in my genes, why did I have cancer?

What were the external factors that led my body to behave in this way?

Some explanations I formulated on my own. Cancer made a scholar out of me.

Some questions will forever remain unanswered.

Cancer didn't make me an oracle.

I did what I had to do so that I could move on. While my answers might not be medically or scientifically proven, they were mine and they helped me move on. Stress caused by various factors, bad relationships, unrealistic pressure I put on myself, poor mental health, depending on pharmaceutical medications for minor ailments and allergies... All of these, I believe, are what led to my body throwing out such an extreme warning signal.

I believe these answers will be different for everyone, because cancer is a different experience for each and every affected person. My own answers helped me want to reduce my stress, live a healthy life, strengthen my immune system, choose my friends more carefully, connect with people who have had a positive impact in my life, and find better (more natural) alternatives to pharmaceutical treatments.

I'll never forget how it all began for me. The shock of it was earth-shattering.

"You have Cancer. Invasive Carcinoma. Stage two, grade 3..." It was June 13th 2016. I was only 32. And the rest was just a blur.

The only thing I remember from meeting Dr H, my breast cancer specialist, is his face - empathetic. The visiting doctor ntext to him had on a stern poker face. They'd asked me if she could sit in for a while. When the news hit me, it didn't matter which doctor was sitting there. In that moment, nothing mattered.

Then there was my husband's face. The colour drained almost completely from his skin. For a few seconds, he went PALE. His lips began to tremble as he looked at me, and that's when I began to weep. For another hour, as the doctors explained everything to me, I cried. I cried inconsolably. I cried with abandon. I remember this because I walked out with a fistful of used tissues bundled up in my hand, into the nurse's room where I cried even more as I broke the news to Baba (my father).

By far, the most difficult thing I did was to break the news to my father, who then bore the responsibility of telling my mother and the rest of the family. I was trembling and crying in the nurse's room, when I decided to call him, they live in Nepal.

Three words, completely unrelated, uttered in a trembling voice and he knew something was wrong.

I asked Baba, "Where are you?"

He said, "Office, *kina- ke bhayo Nanu*?" (Office, why, what's the matter *Nanu*?)

I couldn't control myself. In between trying to hold my breath so I wouldn't break into shuddering sobs, I said, "I'm at the doctors and they said I have cancer." I could hear Baba breathe heavily, and saying, "Shit-shit-shit-shit," over and over again.

This is a man I've never heard curse, especially not in English. Even as I type this, I'm trembling. It still hurts to remember how my father's voice sounded and how he responded to my phone call. I passed the phone to my husband, who was in a slightly better state than me, to handle the rest of the details.

My mother, Mamu, and my aunt, had just taken my grandmother for cataract surgery and were returning home. I thought it wouldn't be a good time to call and speak to her. I asked Baba to go home and to make sure there were people there who could support Mamu when he broke the news to her. I am not sure what happened at home that afternoon, but it certainly isn't something I would like to be told. Some questions are better left unanswered and some emotions should remain unvisited.

Day two was better. Although, I suppose "better" is a strong word. My parents were finding a way to come to the UK, while I was trying to go through the facts and come to terms with the news I had just been given.

You know those five stages of grief that we learn about: denial, anger, bargaining, depression and acceptance? Well, that didn't exactly apply to me. I went through five stages that were all my own. My own turmoil. I even experienced a sixth stage - a stage where I felt a sense of emptiness. I was facing a void; a feeling of not feeling absolutely anything.

I was glad when my parents managed to get a visa to come see me, less than 48 hours after hearing the news that their only child had cancer. All we knew for sure at that moment was that it was in the early stages. The details were still unclear and death was a common theme in all our minds.

Honestly, at that point, my only concern was what would happen to my parents if I didn't make it. I kept blabbing these fears to my husband, who later expressed that he was a little upset that I wasn't more concerned about him. In my opinion, It would certainly impact them harder. The loss of a child is far worse than any other form of grief.

I still regret putting my parents and partner through all that pain and anguish at the time. It's not something I would ever want to go through again.

When adversity hits you, your life gets turned upside down. This particular hardship turned us all inside out as well. It didn't come with a warning label - it never really does, does it? There was no way to prepare for any of it.

At some point, I sat down and thought to myself that only two options lay before me:

1.   Feel sorry for myself and mould my new phase of life with self sympathy and the sympathy donated by others.

2.   Step up to the plate and figure out what I can do now. Discover what comes next and deal with each new experience - good or bad - as it comes.

I chose to explore all the possibilities of moving forward with my head held high, and with my self-esteem and optimism in check. Hopefully, I'd come out of this all with my breasts too - possibly even an upgrade - since the next step for me was a mastectomy.

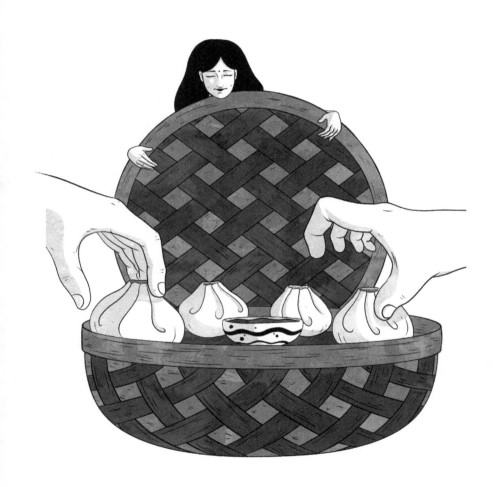

CHAPTER 2

Momo

A PLATFORM FOR COMMUNAL SHARING

Momo is a Nepali dumpling which is generally eaten with a side of tomato achaar - a spicy tomato relish, similar to a salsa in texture, though every self-respecting Nepali will tell you it's not at all similar in taste. It's a versatile food, which can be enjoyed as a snack, for dinner, lunch, or even breakfast. Momo is not just a comfort food for us; it's a symbol of pride that sums up an important part of our identity, reflecting on the highly social aspects of our culture.

An entire family - the women, usually - will use up the entire kitchen space to gather together and make momos. The space becomes an assembly line, conversation corner, and flavour zone all in one! Someone makes the dough, someone else prepares the marinade, and a few others will chop the meat, prep additional ingredients, mix the stuffing together in its glorious entirety, and the rest will fold the dumplings. Anyone who's left will eat.

I think of Momo as a "communal food". That's why it came to mind when I thought about how my cancer experience affected those around me.

I would like to use this chapter as a platform for sharing multiple experiences. First I share an open letter to my friends and families. Then, I asked my husband and my parents to write a note detailing their personal thoughts and feelings on this journey. I have seen and felt most guilty about putting my loved ones through such a difficult time but I have never had the chance - until now - to ask them how they really felt.

As personal as a cancer experience is, the news isn't. My diagnosis affected my family and loved ones. It was hell for me. It was the handbasket for them. We all struggled in different ways.

In desperately grabbing at whatever connections they could find to get an emergency visa from the British embassy, my parents had to discuss what had just happened. Scratching at a wound that's barely healed is painful, and metaphorical wounds are no different. If you're acquainted with a South Asian community, or specifically a Nepali community, news spreads like a wildfire. It's how we band together. It's how we cope.

I wasn't quiet about it. What was there to hide? I didn't exactly announce it publicly on social media but when I spoke to someone, it felt natural to share the details of what had just happened. Later on, "sharing" became a way I overcame the difficulties throughout my journey.

I told my family, my friends, and my peers. In response, I received generous amounts of kind words and support. Unfortunately, because the human condition is flawed, not all responses were appropriate. While everyone meant well, the delivery didn't always land as intended.

As the news of my cancer spread, my inbox, Facebook, and mobile phone began to flood with messages from my nearest and dearest. Messages of courage, hope, and concern filled me with warmth. Those filled with pity and condescension made me absolutely furious. Frankly, some messages were nothing short of offensive. They presented an additional challenge I didn't need. Not only was I working through my own thoughts, but I now had to filter out everyone else's bullcrap too. I had to decipher their meaning and reiterate in my head that they meant well. It was exhausting.

In hindsight, I was (and am) extremely thankful for all the messages and phone calls that came my way. Truly. It was a reminder that people were thinking of me; that they cared enough to show it, no matter how clumsily executed. Any message was better than none at all, which is the route some of my close friends and family chose instead.

Here's an email I drafted in anger (toned down by me a little further down the road). Next time the receivers approach someone who is grieving, they might just be able to understand and edit their messages of "support".

Dear Family, Friends, Loved Ones,

Thank you for all the messages that have flooded my mailbox, phone, and social media. I really appreciate those who took the time to write to me. I am sorry for not replying earlier or not answering your calls. As it happens, I was trying to convert my disbelief and grief into the ability to deal with the daily battle of acceptance.

I know that every message sent to me was delivered with an honest heart and the love you have for me.

I have realised that even the best intentions can come off as hurtful or inappropriate. Some messages I can now read and laugh about, but in my moments of pain, they weren't at all comforting.

Let me have been your guinea pig. Your final chance to say the wrong things. I don't hold the things you've said to me against you. I've learned from them. It's only right that you do too. Let me give you some tips on how to deal with this better if (God forbid) you find yourself in a similar situation again.

The biggest no-no on my list is giving someone advice if you haven't been through cancer or been a caretaker of a cancer patient yourself. Going to the hospital because you fainted from a stomach bug is NOT the same thing as being rushed to the ER with neutropenic sepsis. You cannot draw parallels to try and show that you know what someone else is going through. In fact, as someone with zero experience in this situation, you're not drawing a parallel. You're drawing an octagon.

All you can do is give love, ask me how I am doing, make me laugh, make my meals, send me cards and letters that make my day, and hug me tight and kiss me to tell me that you care. Just make me feel normal. I'm still a person. I am not the disease.

There are culturally sensitive terms, and then there are cancer-ally sensitive sentences. This could probably be applied to the wider genera of people going through chronic medical conditions. (But I'm no expert, so I suggest you bother to check with them first!) Though bear in mind, "I just don't know what to say," is better than not saying anything at all.

What I have listed below are some sentences that are not in any way made up, even though it may sound like it. I just have a good memory. Also, I kept a diary because my "good memory" isn't actually all that great.

WTF: "You are so beautiful, how can this happen to you?"

Thoughts: Yes, because tiny tumour cells are not only aggressively intrusive but also only attack ugly people? This comment made me realise how stupid and unaware people are about cancer. Cancer is on the rise, that's a fact. Many of us will encounter (or be close to) someone who is currently battling cancer or has done so in the past. Maybe people should make an effort to learn more about what someone is going through before saying something so ridiculous.

WTF: "It's your past life's sins. The universe is trying to tell you something. You have to accept it in this life, so it won't carry over into your next life."

Thoughts: Can I please deal with this in THIS life, and not give a rats ass about a past life. Are you really telling me that I deserved this BECAUSE of the consequences of a life I am not even aware of? I should just accept my fate because a version of me that may or may not have existed is responsible for this hot mess? Blaming my current self and desperately searching for answers isn't difficult enough, right?

WTF: "Do you think this happened to you because you didn't have a baby sooner?"

Thoughts: Have you lost your damn mind? With absolutely no medical proof, you're telling me that people who have babies when they are younger are exempt from a potential cancer diagnosis. You're pointing the finger at women everywhere who have a right to choose when, where, or whether to have babies at all. You're lathering on the guilt without a second's pause. I've met young women who, at the tender age of 19 were NOT baby factories, and still had been diagnosed with cancer. Keep your pseudo-medical nonsense to yourself.

WTF: "Oh! Cancer is not as bad as it used to be before, and you have the good type of cancer."

Thoughts: Yeah, sure, I'm lucky. Thanks for enlightening me. This is a walk in the park. I might as well have the flu. The Good Cancer - it's like an unreturnable gift I didn't want. Merely an inconvenience. I should totally be the one to make the compromise and be less upset because I wasn't heaped with the Bad Cancer.

WTF: "I've always wanted to shave my head, you got to do it."

Thoughts: Listen here, Fashion Police, this wasn't my choice. I didn't shave my head because I felt like it. It was a traumatic experience. My hair FELL OUT. It scarpered, disappeared, abandoned me, and didn't return until the very end of my treatment cycle. This included my eyelashes and eyebrows. It wasn't a fashion statement. It was a reminder that nothing would ever be the same.

WTF: "I know how you feel, I hate hospitals. This one time I broke my arm and had to be rushed into the ER..."

Thoughts: You know what, if you can't see how wrong this is, I can't help you.

WTF: "You are so brave, you are so strong."

Thoughts: Bet you didn't expect to see this one here. It's a weird one, I'll be honest. It all depends on what stage of the cancer journey this was mentioned at or how much you actually know about what I have gone through. At the beginning of my journey, do you really know what I'm facing and how I'm going to deal with it? If you're saying this to me after really making the effort to find out how I dealt with cancer, it's kinda nice to hear. You have a 50/50 chance of this comment falling flat, so maybe find a better way to phrase what you're trying to say. After all, a cancer patient has two choices: be strong and brave or face death. So, you're not really saying much.

WTF: "At least you will live."

Thoughts: Hey, Oracle, how do you know? Don't diminish my experience because it makes it easier for you to deal with. Yes, I was diagnosed in the somewhat early stages BUT there are no guarantees. Cancer treatment isn't an exact science. I didn't need anyone making me out to be some kind of hypochondriac. For someone who has never faced cancer, either personally or through someone else, this comment just isn't justifiable.

WTF: "You should try this diet. I read about it online," or, "Eat this, I know of someone who healed herself by just eating this."

Thoughts: I get it. People become overwhelmed by the idea of giving ideas and tips to help. It's not unappreciated but it is misguided. My parents and I both fell victim to this when we went out of our way to find soursop, a fruit which is not very easily available in London. I also went to great lengths to add moringa powder to

EVERYTHING I ate. It's great to eat healthy; to eat fruits and vegetables, and to incorporate more spices in every meal. It helps in so many ways but it's not going to heal cancer. You're not going to be able to provide your loved ones with specific foods that will take their illness or pain away. You also don't know how certain foods will interact. Despite all the advice given, my body rejected the soursop. No miracle cure there.

Those are just a few of the gems I jotted down. Do you see how your words have an effect on the person you're trying to help?

Never ever, if you haven't been through this process, make suggestions on treatment, diet, or wonder cures. It is never helpful to anyone. Trust me, I did try anything and everything. Adding to an already lengthy list doesn't make it better.

Yes, there are people who believe solely in natural therapy. Yes, a few people have miraculously healed themselves with either food or a specific herb. Unfortunately, this doesn't work for everyone. There is a reason medical professionals are there to give you expert advice.

I tried hard to see the good side to every message but I found it difficult to accept words of wisdom from people who just don't have a clue. Cancer is still the same cancer it was when it was first discovered. Sure, medical science has helped us understand it a little better, treatments have progressed a lot, and the survival rate is much higher now than it was many years ago. That doesn't mean it isn't a scary beast for someone who is new to it all, like I was.

Cancer is a complex condition. My doctors and nurses constantly reminded me that no two cases are the same - ever! So, when you're reaching out to someone who is dealing with their own battle, try to do so with caution and curiosity, rather than know-it-all advice. Offering advice is a habit for so many of us, one that is worth breaking. If you grew up in a South Asian culture, giving advice is synonymous with helping someone who is feeling unwell, so it can be particularly difficult to avoid. Try anyway.

Ask for and respect, without personal prejudice, the comments of someone going through cancer. The urge to help is undeniably strong. But if you're not actually being helpful, you're adding undue pressure. I, personally, didn't want help from anyone other than my parents and husband. I often turned down offers from my friends, cousins, and relatives. The fact that they didn't push it any further was a huge weight off my shoulders and helped me more than they know.

For those who said very little but said the right thing, you gave me the courage to face cancer and to overcome any insecurities. The love and positive energy that you gave me helped me change my overall outlook on cancer.

Here are some of the statements that were comforting:

> "I love you, please let me know if I can do anything."

> "I'm sorry this happened to you."

> "I'm sorry you have to go through this."

> "If you ever need to talk, please let me know, I am always here for you."

Those random messages that said, "Thinking about you, sending you a big hug," those were the best.

I appreciated it when people made me feel normal by suggesting a coffee or going for a movie. I always tried my best to join when I was up for it.

When people would still call me to tell me some of the problems they were facing, I felt valued. I felt a sense of normalcy. After all, I am still the same person and, in any situation, I will remain a friend, cousin, or niece.

Always remember that you can be a big part of someone's healing process, like it was for me. Your messages taught me resilience, gave me patience, and showed me how much I am loved.

Thank you for that.

A Note From my Husband:

As my wife - who I'm very proud of - suggested in this chapter, what a cancer patient feels is very personal to them. What their carer feels, is a personal experience that stands on its own too. On a daily basis, they go through a variety of emotions. Every day can be great, crap, exhausting, happy, nerve-racking, challenging, and hopeful. The challenge lies in figuring out how to handle it and putting up a genuine smile when it feels like your world is collapsing around your ears. Genuine. That's the key.

I run a tech start-up in London. It's a lot like having a baby - one that demands all the attention you can muster. Like a baby poops and sleeps, a start-up has shitty days and good ones. What makes it worth it, is knowing that one day it will mature into something great.

Managing a business in its infancy is difficult enough. Trying to balance it all when your wife is going through the emotional, mental, and physical ringer… Well, that feels borderline impossible.

I'm not ashamed to admit that I struggled on days when I was alone with Sue and had to manage everything. I often had to bring my laptop to the hospital so that I could do some work when Sue was asleep. I'm blessed to have a fantastic team at Goodman Lantern who supported me through the journey.

There is one incident on this journey that I'll never forget. It was Sue's 4th round of chemo and the doctors had started a new drug. I was told that if she felt feverish, I should rush her to hospital immediately. One evening after her session, and when my in-laws were on their way from London to Kathmandu, Sue felt severely unwell. No questions asked, I rushed her to the ER. During our drive in the Uber, she was totally unresponsive. At some points, it felt like she was looking right through me. Either she wasn't there, or in her mind, I wasn't there. Neither scenario was a good one.

When we reached the hospital, tests were done immediately. Her white blood cell counts were 0.4. They should have been in the upper single digits; at least 7 or higher. Doctors were clear to point out that this could be fatal. This could be it for her, for us, for our future.

That night, I left the hospital at 1am after finding out she had neutropenic sepsis, a serious unknown infection. I wasn't allowed to stay the night. It was the longest walk home I'd ever experienced. When I reached home, my eyes fell on the picture we'd taken in Austria just a few months earlier. That was my breaking point, and I couldn't stop the tears from rolling down my cheeks.

That was the day I realised that what I wanted more than anything was "us". It occurred to me that life is short. We should value every minute we spend together. Some people say cancer breaks families, I believe it brought us together.

There are multiple strategies I could have used to cope with it all. I know where my strengths lie, so I thought of it as a project. Something that needed smart management. My mission was to help Sue get through it all with minimal amounts of stress for her. I developed a routine to ask her how she felt every couple of hours and listened to her when she complained. Earlier on, I wanted to give her my thoughts but quickly I realised what she needed was someone to hear her.

There were days when I felt like there was nothing I could do to help her. I imagine that is how most caregivers feel. Honestly, though, just being there for her, listening to her, and helping her with food, toilet visits, and other daily tasks felt good.

I kept suggesting that Sue think about the entire treatment process as a countdown. Break it down into 6 chemos and 15 radiotherapies. Instead of thinking of it as a never-ending cycle, think, "We are 3 chemos down, only 3 to go." We needed to find small reasons to celebrate the progress she was making.

There were also days when I just couldn't deal with things. That's when my in-laws being around really helped. I love my food and once a week I would go to enjoy a greasy burger and beer. It was 'me' time and all I needed was to feel normal again.

Coping mechanisms help foster a sense of normalcy. I needed to recharge and boost my inner strength levels. How else could I be there for Sue?

Self-care is an important part of the journey for the carer.

A Note From my Parents

Although I had requested that my mother and father write separate notes, my mother couldn't bring herself to reopen those emotional wounds. She didn't want to revisit that pain again and I didn't want to force her. She said she would help my father with his note, but later found out that even as my dad read out the note to her, she almost couldn't listen to it all again - it's just too raw, and I understand that.

She called me on Viber while I was at the office in a meeting. I was aware that she had gone to get her reports, so I already knew I had to step outside and answer her call.

As soon as I heard, "Baba, my report is positive," I felt like I had just fallen off a roof. My colleagues noticed my reaction and figured something was wrong. They came to console me. "Baba, don't worry. It's in an early stage and I'm at the best hospital in the world. The doctors have said I will make a full recovery."

At the time, Suvekchya's mother was with her sister and her mother, Suvekchya's grandmother, who was being escorted back home after a cataract surgery. Knowing this, Suvekchya told me she had not spoken to her mother yet. She decided that I should head home and tell her mother there, while she continued with her appointment at the doctor's office.

By the time I reached home and told my wife, Suvekchya and Raj were home. We were panicking and were not sure how to handle ourselves but I still remember how calm and positive our daughter was. Her strength in that moment made us all calmer and able to discuss the situation at hand.

We were in Nepal at the time and didn't have a VISA for the UK. We wanted to get to our daughter as soon as possible. In no matter of time, our close friends and family found out and flooded our house to keep us company. Many of them used their connections to contact the British Embassy in India, because all the VISA applications are done by VFS in Nepal, and sent to India to be processed.

Meanwhile, keeping in mind that the VISA might take some time, we discussed options for Suvekchya's treatment in either Singapore or Thailand, so she could be closer to home. In case the paperwork didn't come through, she would need to be closer by so we would be able to see her more easily. But our son-in-law stayed level-headed and convinced us that the VISA would not be a problem in such circumstances. Additionally, the hospital that she would be receiving treatment at is one of the best cancer research centres in the UK.

We soon flew to Delhi, India to get our emergency VISA. From there, my wife and I took the longest nine-hour flight to London. We had no idea where we were flying, or why and for how long - we were in shock. It felt like we were in limbo. My wife and I kept looking at each other every now and then without having a word to say to each other. It just felt like our world was coming to an end.

When we landed at Heathrow Airport and saw our daughter and son in law, we felt a big sigh of relief - at least momentarily. In our taxi ride back to their house, our daughter explained the entire treatment process. In between, Raj was trying to ease our nerves.

When we eventually got home, we had time to discuss every little detail. It was a long drive back. We were almost in tears when our daughter said something I will never forget, "It is what it is, *Baba* and *Mamu*. Talking about it further won't make it go away or help anyone. It'll only make us panic more. So from now on, we will not dwell on this any more but focus on my treatment and moving forward."

Her words were powerful. They helped us find the positive attitude we needed to support her.

During the next few months, we were impressed to see Raj's patience and the way he took care of our daughter. This was when we realised that God really gave us a great son-in-law. He was her true support and strength; an example of a good life partner. There were only four of us in a foreign country with no other support than each other.

There were many sleepless nights thinking about Suvekchya's cancer, all the hospital visits, upcoming surgery, and other treatments. Everything was daunting to think about. What gave us the strength to overcome that was our daughter's power and strong-will. Her conversations were always positive; always thankful for finding out about her cancer at an early stage and being in the right place at the right time.

I still remember the day of her surgery. We had about 21 relatives, friends, and family friends who came to be with us.

The pain of seeing your daughter go through the surgery and chemotherapy was absolutely unbearable for us. Raj's constant support and Suvekchya's strength, willpower, and positivity made us really appreciate our daughter's capacity to fight all of this. She was a support to us and we to her.

Thinking about all her suffering and agony, we wished we could take it away with us. There was never a day when our daughter complained, cried, or showed us that she was suffering. Nevertheless, we understood and saw the hardship she went through mentally and physically. As a parent, there is nothing worse than seeing your child suffer and not being able to do anything about it.

To be able to overcome all of this and lead a healthy life, we are forever grateful to the hospital, doctor, nurses, and all the support from our loved ones. We also can't thank our dear son-in-law enough for being patient and taking such good care of our only child. For this we are eternally grateful.

It's undeniable that cancer has an enormous impact on loved ones. It may be a lonely disease but the ripple effect is quite substantial. I decided not to show too much emotion throughout the process. It's a part of my personality that I wasn't going to let cancer take from me. My willingness to persevere through this without showing any pain or suffering was so deeply ingrained that I chose to put a smile on my face, no matter what.

I chose not to complain so that it would not affect my family. And it worked, mostly. They were relieved to see me happy and overcoming the beast. On the other hand, there were times when I could not mask my feelings. When I was vomiting, or had a physical allergic reaction, or my face and body swelled as my heart began to give up, these were things I could not hide. This is when families feel helpless. They feel that they can't stop their wife or daughter or friend from suffering. This is something I will never be able to understand - it's a wholly different struggle to my own that's caused by the same condition.

Communication is so important. I realise this now more than ever. If I'd been able to talk to someone beforehand - if someone had shared their journey with me - maybe I'd have been able to deal with certain things differently.

I'll leave you with this thought as I close off this chapter:

> Please talk to your daughter, your wife, or mother about breast cancer. Getting to know your body is the best way to know when something isn't right. Look at your body, feel your skin, appreciate your entire self. Encourage each other to speak more about cancer, know more about cancer, and learn what it is. Being aware is what you can do now. Start straight away.

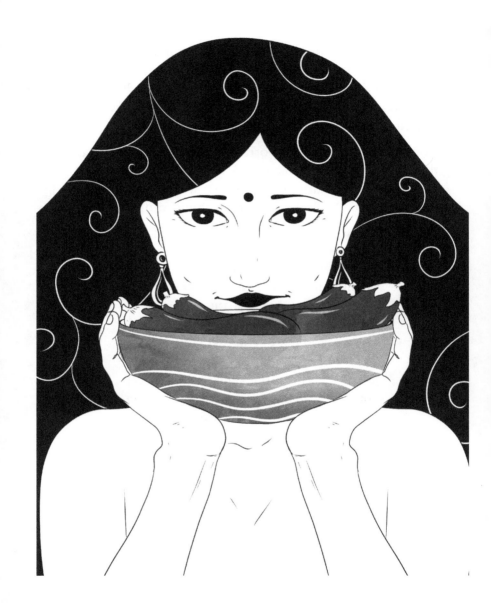

CHAPTER 3

Bhanta ko Bharta

SURGERY AND RECONSTRUCTION

Bhanta is "Aubergine" in Nepali. Bhanta ko Bharta, more popularly known as "Baigan ka Bharta" in India, is a simple dish made of grilled aubergine that is smashed with aromatics and spices.

While the aubergine is being grilled, generally over a gas hob or in an oven, the insides become soft and smushy while the outer shape is totally deformed. When I saw my right breast for the first time, post mastectomy, that's all I could see. The anti-aubergine. A brinjal blob.

Surgery was the first step in my treatment plan: a complete right mastectomy, followed by reconstruction. Because I was still young, my doctors recommended that I do a reconstruction. At the time, it really didn't seem important. I wanted to be cancer-free. It didn't matter whether I could satisfactorily fill a bra or not.

I went along with the suggestion but didn't think much of it. Although, admittedly, when I did find the time to process it all eventually, a new set of boobs was pretty exciting. Fake boobs. Foobs. *Bodaciousness* was on the horizon. It's

31

difficult not to be excited about something like that! With all the heavy stuff I still needed to process, this was a little gift to lighten the gloom.

When I first began to fantasise about the reconstruction, I pictured myself as a Victoria's Secret model. In my head, it was all firm perkiness and low cut dresses. Maybe a Baywatch bounce in a sexy swimsuit. My imaginary future rack was truly enviable.

Back down on Earth, my surgeon asked me if I would prefer my reconstruction size to be the same as before. Would I perhaps like to go a few sizes bigger? My jaw dropped at this point - who would have thought the Baywatch daydream was actually a possibility?

Unlike the West that has an obsession with large breasts, South Asian culture is a little different. Culture aside, it's really not my scene either - not on my own body, anyway. Before my diagnosis, I was already blessed with a beautiful body, breasts and all. I jokingly told the plastic surgeon to "go smaller". I received a hearty chuckle for my stoicism.

Breast enlargement is a familiar concept to most people - it's not the taboo procedure it may once have been. Women are free to take control of their bodies and adjust them surgically to their preference. In most cases, boob jobs are thought to be a fairly sexy bodily upgrade.

Spoiler alert: reconstructive surgery after a mastectomy is anything but glamorous. I imagine that reconstruction after a bilateral mastectomy is doubly unglamorous.

Growing up, I had never had any kind of incision on my body. No stitches or major injuries. Maybe a trip or two to the ENT, the occasional tooth filling, the rare x-ray... Hospitals, thus far, hadn't meant surgery of any kind.

As weird as it sounds, going through the details beforehand had me feeling both terrified and excited. I would be experiencing general anaesthetic for the first time. After all the stories I'd heard about people on morphine - and no shortage of YouTube videos, I wondered what secrets would escape from my drugged-out self.

On the flip-side, I was scared. A part of my body was going to be forcibly removed. This wasn't a reversible procedure. It felt like part of what defined my femininity was about to be ripped from me. My breasts - any woman's breasts - are part of what clearly defines the physical feminine form.

There was a week between finding out I had cancer and the surgery. That's not much time to process. We had parents coming over to help us, relatives and friends visiting, and a fair amount of bustle going on all the time. I didn't have much time to think things over.

Maybe that was a good thing. I didn't have the luxury of dwelling on the unknown.

I had to undergo a few tests before the procedure, including injecting a small dose of radiation around the surgery site. When illuminated under a special light, this would help the surgeons see how far the cancer had spread. Apparently, cancer cells absorb radiation very well, so they are easily visible during the surgery.

I was hesitant about this particular step. I expressed how uncomfortable I was about injecting radiation inside my body. I mean, I know all about Chernobyl... What about the side effects? How would I get rid of the radiation later on?

As it turns out, hopping on a flight to Cordoba, Spain a month previously had exposed me to more radiation than the injection would. Thanks for ruining air travel...

After receiving this little nugget of information, I decided to keep quiet and let the professionals do what they do best.

I remember acting all cool, taking selfies in my hospital gown, showing off the wrist-band and cannula before my surgery. When I was called in, reality hit and I began to tremble. What if I didn't wake up afterwards?

Walking through the seemingly endless corridor through the surgical section of the hospital, decked out in my blue gown and white anti-embolism socks, I began to cry. Luckily, my husband and parents didn't see me this way.

Finally, I was met with a familiar face - Dr H. His bow tie was clearly visible through his surgical gown and he was armed with a comforting smile. When he asked me how I was doing, I had a one-word answer: "Scared."

His simple response of, "Of course," was a comfort on its own. He didn't need to say more as he held my hand and guided me towards the next step. Empathy is all a person really needs in situations like these, and I was grateful for it.

The anaesthetist asked me to tell him about my favourite dessert.

I got all the way to, "Tirami-," before I was out. I sometimes wonder if my unconscious self ever managed to finish off the, "- su."

The surgery lasted just over two hours. When I woke up, I felt worse than I ever had, or ever imagined I could. I was shivering. It felt like I had been shocked. I was IN shock. The pain was indescribable.

When I woke up, the nurse who was next to me said, "The surgery was good, you will feel better soon. Your surgeon will be here soon." It seemed like such a mundane statement, when the world was very clearly ending. The pain was so bad, I couldn't even speak. The foggy after-effects of the anaesthesia weren't much help either, but I managed to smile and mumble a "thank you".

The nurse realised I was very cold and put a few more blankets over me. I thought about my parents and my husband but they were not in the recovery room. An hour or two later, I was moved into a ward. This is where I stayed for the next few days, supported by the morphine pen next to my bed and my fellow *breasties* (a term often used to refer to other girls who've had either a single or bi-lateral mastectomy).

The day I dreaded most was only 12 days after my surgery. It was the day I would see my scars and my new right breast. By then, I had read a ton of stuff online. I'd quickly learned that I shouldn't be alone for it. It would be an emotional revelation. Although I'd educated myself beforehand, it also dawned on me that my natural organ had been replaced with a blob of silicon packaged in either cow or pig skin. I didn't dare ask for specifics on precisely which animal had donated the extra fat to my body.

Up until that point, body image had never been a major problem for me. I was comfortable in my own skin. I've been blessed with great genes. I'm a good height and I had always had an abundance of silky hair. My skin was clear and, frankly, my breasts and ass were pretty good too. Sure, I had a few lapses (especially during my teen years) where I wished for longer, straighter, or curlier hair, or skin that was a shade or two darker or lighter. But ultimately, I was pretty self-confident and comfortable.

I understood why some people would have insecurities. Yet, I had never fully understood why anyone would be ashamed of their body. I didn't really love my body - because we are never really permitted to think of our bodies in that way - but I didn't hate it either. All of this changed after my surgery. Honestly, it still continues to have an impact on the way I see myself.

The implant, regardless of how great the surgeon is, isn't easy to get used to. I'm not sure you ever really do get completely used to it. Once the mammary glands and muscles around the area are completely removed, your breasts don't look and feel the same ever again. I only had one done, so I have a constant battle with how different my pair looks.

One thing to prepare yourself for after a reconstruction (if you are having one) is that it will take a long time for you to get used to the new fake boob (fondly referred to as a "foob") - both physically and mentally. For me, at first it felt heavy and uncomfortable.

Soon, I was greeted with the very real (rather disappointing, at the time) truth: two absolutely different looking chesticles. One breast was in-sync with the laws of gravity. The other was trying its best to greet the moon and stars. My new boob was heavy and uncomfortable; a weird new attachment that wasn't playing along with my hopes or expectations.

For the longest time, this un-boob of mine was such a sore point that I nicknamed it "Joker's Smile."

You're probably acquainted with Joker from the Batman storyline. You've seen his face. Those deep scars on his cheeks, clumsily masked by a grotesque crescent-smile of bright red lipstick; the garish crimson colour seeping into the haggard creases around his lips. That's what my scar looked like to me; going from left to right, the long crescent shaped across my new breasts.

After my reconstruction, I had to wear a special sort of sports bra for six to eight weeks. The recovery time felt like years. The really terrible granny bra made it feel like forever. I longed for the joyous moment when I could wear a proper, ladylike bra again. Unfortunately, when I got to that point, something just didn't fit right. The inconsiderate blob had struck again.

While my left breast grew or shrank as I lost or gained weight, my right foob stayed the same. Great.

A breast implant is like a memory foam mattress. Over time, it "learns" to take on your body shape. It takes my foob some time to settle into the shape of any particular bra. Like kinetic sand readjusting itself but much slower. I needed to adjust to the bizarre behaviour of my new appendage. Every time I put on a different type of bra, my boob needs some time to get into the game. Poor thing just needs to be left alone to do its thing. And this shapeshifting nonsense isn't just limited to my underwear. When I sleep on my belly, the first few minutes are exceedingly uncomfortable, but within 5-10 minutes, good ol' Fooby finds her place.

These personal details might seem a little overwhelming, or maybe even inappropriate to some. I want you to know that I'm not throwing a pity party. People who are unaware of these things need to gain an understanding of what a cancervivor goes through. This information isn't readily available out there.

Getting used to a new "self" is a difficult process. We all go through something different. In sharing my story, I hope to shed some light on how deeply personal this all is. Cancer isn't purely medical. It's emotional and mental too.

Before now, before this life-altering experience, my breasts - or anyone else's - weren't an appropriate topic of discussion. Not within my family or culture, anyway.

Now, it's somehow acceptable to discuss my breasts - or lack thereof, on the one side. I can freely speak about my reduced chances of reproducing due to chemotherapy. Aunties and uncles who I could never have spoken to about this stuff before are listening to me and sympathizing with me. Suddenly, all of this was the topic of discussion during group skype chats, at dinner, and over drinks at the bar.

Why, in our culture, do we wait for a life-altering experience before we can be open about things that matter? Why do we wait for someone to be knocking at Death's door before we can openly discuss diseases, reproductive organs, and 'intimate' body parts?

I think we should talk about all of it as a family. As parents, as friends, as teachers to students... Maybe this will help younger generations to stop body shaming, and to understand what's normal and what is not.

Now that I've had time to adjust, I am happy with my *kuche-ko bhanta*. Anyone who's seen me can't even tell that I've had reconstructive breast surgery. I've been blessed with the most talented surgeons who have now done not only one, but two reconstructive surgeries on me.

I am grateful for what I have and who I am. I feel confident enough to make fun of myself, share my experiences, and to tell the world that I am finally happy with my body.

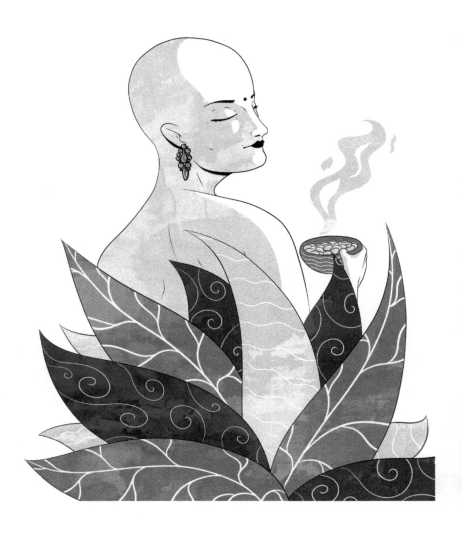

CHAPTER 4

Swan Puka

CHEMOTHERAPY

"Swan Puka" basically translates to stuffed and fried goat's lungs. It might not be the most appealing flavour profile to a Westernised palate but, just like gizzards, lungs are a delicacy in many cultures.

When making Swan Puka, the lungs are thoroughly cleaned and then, using a tube, stuffed with spices. Once the lungs have been filled, they are cut into pieces and fried. It's surprisingly tasty.

I draw the analogy to Swan Puka because I felt very much like a live version of the goat, having high doses of medication stuffed into my veins. The tubes may be tinier but that doesn't make the experience any more enjoyable. Each chemotherapy "stuffing" session took at least 2-4 hours depending on the type of drugs they were inserting. Much like the spices were meant to make the goat taste better, my own stuffing process was meant to make me healthier. I heavily doubt that this made me any tastier...

For most cancer patients, the treatment process involves chemotherapy. The drug (or combination of drugs) kills all rapidly growing cells in your body. It gets rid of not only the cancer cells, which generally divide and grow much faster than normal cells, but also other healthy and useful cells within the body. Chemo can be given orally as a tablet or through injection.

Beyond a shadow of a doubt, this was the most difficult, painful, and traumatic phase of my life. It was darkness.

If you've had chemotherapy, or sat through someone's first chemo consultation with them, you'll know that you sign your life away. That's how detrimental chemo is to your body. Yet, it's required. A double-edged sword.

I remember reading through the five-page paper and feeling like I was signing something truly dangerous. Don't quote me word for word but this document basically stated that, if I died during chemo (or ended up with permanent organ damage) the oncologist, doctors, and medical team would not be held responsible.

I went home with a copy of that deathly document and listed all the organs the chemo would affect. And, it was pretty much everything. From your eyes to your stomach, your kidneys, heart, liver, and hair.

I now understand why so many people are against chemotherapy. At the time, I, like many others, didn't have much knowledge about chemo. I knew what it was, but had no idea how insane its effects could be.

Honestly, if you haven't experienced it firsthand, or taken care of someone who has, you seriously don't have a clue. You simply don't understand the depth of its physical or emotional impact.

All six rounds of my chemo - a combination of FEC-T drugs - were done intravenously. The first three months were a combination of Fluorouracil, Epirubicin, and

Cyclophosphamide (FEC). The last three were Docetaxel (Taxotere or T).

My very first experience of chemo seemed to be a pleasant one. I walked with my mum and husband to the hospital in high spirits. My father on the other hand was back home with his family.

The Universe clearly believed that our family was strong enough to handle two traumatic experiences at the same time. My dad had to stay back in Nepal to perform the last rites for his father who had passed away only two days before my parents scheduled their flight to London. My paternal grandfather passed away in his sleep, after suffering major kidney damage and undergoing multiple dialyses. My father was torn. He wanted to be with his child for her first chemo but as the eldest son, he had a duty to perform. More importantly, he needed time to be with his mother and family and to mourn this loss.

With a heavy heart but a strong determination, it was time to start beating this thing that had taken an unwelcome hold of my body. I was called straight inside, so I had no time to feel daunted by the waiting room. The nurse struggled to find a good vein initially but she got there eventually.

During the first hour, the nurse had to sit beside me to press the syringe. One of the medications was intensely strong and had to be physically inserted - squeezed - regularly. It burned a little but there was saline in the same catheter so the medicine could be diluted to make it more bearable for the body. The process took about three hours and I was back home in time for lunch. I ate a massive meal and went to sleep, thinking to myself, *"This is not bad at all, and hey, I ate a big meal. I have an appetite, so what on earth are people talking about, what side effects?"*

An hour later, I woke up with the most uncomfortable nauseated feeling. I rushed to the toilet to orally relieve myself of my lunch. This continued for the next six hours. I vomited almost every hour, by the clock.

This was just the start.

I had always had tiny veins. It runs in the family. I have seen my mother go off to get blood taken and come back with three of four veins poked to pieces. For chemo, you need a strong vein that does not collapse. The medication is intense and needs veins that will be able to maintain their integrity while being injected. My veins burned and itched while I sat patiently for hours. They could only use my left arm because I'd had a mastectomy on the right. Because some of my lymph nodes were extracted, I will not be allowed to take blood from my right hand for the rest of my life. This is due to an increased risk of Lymphedema, they say.

To combat my tiny vein issue, I put my left arm under a warm heater, jumped up and down, and drank a gallon of water just so my veins would be easy to find. The first half an hour was always a serious struggle between my veins and the nurse. They would never agree which round of poking to give up on. The nurse often took it personally and it always resulted in the entire oncology team trying to help me.

There were moments when we almost had to resort to looking for a vein in my legs but, somehow before that moment of desperation, something would work. The doctors recommended that I have a PICC (peripherally inserted central catheter) line put in. The PICC line is a thin, soft, very long catheter that they inserted into a vein in my left arm. As is usually the case, the vein they chose was one that carries blood directly to the heart. The end of the catheter was covered and cleaned regularly by nurses, making sure that the open end wouldn't get infected. With this addition, my chemo sessions were free from fruitless jabs.

It must have been my fourth chemo - third with a PICC - when one of my regular "chemo buddies" mentioned that her PICC line had a clot. Although I didn't have any symptoms, her announcement made me curious enough to mention it to the nurse. To set my mind at ease, she decided to send me for a scan. Lo and behold, I had a clot too. The PICC line was immediately removed and I had to go back to regular IV.

This unnecessary complication also meant that I had to give myself an anticoagulant injection every day for the next six months. Every day. While anticoagulants come in tablet form too, I was unable to take them due to the ongoing chemotherapy. There are no shortcuts, no easy roads to travel when it comes to cancer treatment.

While I was on blood thinners, it was made clear that cuts and bruises were to be avoided at all costs. I would bleed more than normal and bruise very easily. Unfortunately (or fortunately), my mother was with me when the doctors made this announcement. From that moment, she became hawk-like in her efforts to keep me away from anything even vaguely sharp - knives included. At mealtimes, she would take the knife away from me, cut my food into bite-size pieces, and leave me with only a fork. I felt like a three-year-old again. Every time I used the oven or grabbed a pair of scissors, I was investigated and interrogated.

This went on for six months, until I turned 33.

In the beginning, it was impossible to leave home because, at 6 pm, it was time for the injection. My schedule revolved around that stupid injection. I soon became comfortable with jabbing myself. At some point, I decided to carry it in my purse, excuse myself around 6 pm, go to the ladies and do the needful. Towards the end, my confidence level rose to 100%. At one point, when I was at dinner with friends in an extremely crowded restaurant, I didn't want to go to the trouble of looking for a toilet. So, I pardoned myself, lifted my top, lowered my trousers to my waistline and jabbed as I continued to eat my starter.

Guess whose fear of needles soon disappeared?

T, or Docetaxel, is the Mother of All Evil. All the three rounds I had, resulted in being rushed to the ER; twice to critical care and once to the resuscitation area. Both instances started with a high fever. Fever during chemo is like a massive, brightly illuminated danger sign, flashing in capital letters. Fever means only one thing: infection. Infection during chemo is a one-way ticket to the afterlife. There are days when your white blood cells are at their weakest, unable to fight any external or internal infections. At that point, even a common cold can kill you. I was instructed to rush straight to the emergency room anytime I had a fever. All three times I headed to the ER, my fever was super high.

The first time, it was a serious case of neutropenic sepsis and the other was an unknown infection, when the round of chemo resulted in my heart almost giving up; beating irregularly. During the first case, my parents had just left for the airport. My mother was booked in for her own surgery back home - so she was heading home to rest and recover. I said goodbye to them and went to bed. I woke up a few hours later to realise that my spine and bones weren't working. I could not sit up or move.

I managed to call my husband, who was in the other room. I asked him to check if I had a fever, and I did. He called an Uber and we rushed to the ER. While on the road, he kept asking me how I was doing and was met with a blank stare. I recall nothing of this car ride. Within a few hours, I was informed that I had sepsis and I was severely neutropenic. The usual white blood cell count should have been at around 7-10 units. Mine was sitting at 0.4.

I was moved into a separate room and put in isolation. For the next five days, I was constantly on fluids and the nurses and doctors had to wear special aprons, masks, and gloves when they came to see me. This applied to any visitors too, though they were allowed to visit me only after the third day, once I was out of danger.

The second episode wasn't as bad as the first. It was only an ER visit with prescribed antibiotics and a follow-up. The third time was indeed the charm. By this time, I had lost all my hair, including my eyebrows and eyelashes. Mr. Fever came to visit at around 3 am, when I woke up to go to the loo.

I had to wake my husband and my parents, who were in the next room. By the time I was taken to the hospital, my face and body had swollen to the point that I was unrecognisable. My face looked like someone had drawn eyes, a mouth, and a nose on a balloon. I was kept in the resuscitation ward with machines hooked up all over my chest. I was constantly being monitored by nurses. My fever finally went away after about 10 hours. We had absolutely no idea of where the infection was festering. I spent two days in hospital and was discharged with a sackful of antibiotics. As if I didn't have enough medication coursing through me already.

I had gained a significant amount of weight (around 10kg), lost all my hair, eyebrows and eyelashes, gained another chin and an extra layer around my neck. My nails began to look a little ragged and so did my teeth. I wore looser clothes because nothing else fit me and I was in no position to go shopping. I often covered myself with a big sleeping bag-sized poncho. The side effects of the steroids and other medications were a bit much for my body.

One incident I remember rather fondly is when I was waiting outside a supermarket, for my husband to return, a lady approached me to give me a fiver. She must have thought I was homeless. Even then, I could see the humour in the situation.

Here are a few more of my not-so-fondly remembered side-effects that I would like to share with you:

HAIR

Alopecia areata, more commonly referred to as "patchy hair loss", is almost inevitable when you subject your body to chemotherapy, especially if it is FEC-T. When I found out I was going to lose my hair, I booked an appointment at a hair salon for the very next day. I had them cut off 13 inches of my hair and I donated it to Locks of Love.

I was advised to give the cold cap a chance, to preserve what was left of my hair. And I did. This system cools the scalp by narrowing the blood vessels beneath the skin, reducing the amount of medication that reaches the hair follicles. With very little chemo reaching your head, the hair may be less likely to fall out.

The surplus hair on my head was too much for the cool cap to handle. So, every morning I woke up to bundles of hair all over my pillow. Any time I ran my hand through my hair, it came out in chunks, leaving my head patchy and unkempt. It was an absolute horror to deal with every day. I still have to block out memories of the time I tried to wash my hair, against the doctors' recommendations - fistfuls of my formerly glorious tresses littering the shower floor.

One early morning, I woke up to the uncomfortable feeling of hair all over my face, neck, and body. To my dismay, the hair from my head had fallen out even more. It was pouring from the pillow to my sheets. A seemingly endless river of my precious mane. I had had enough! I went to the bathroom, sat in the bathtub, and began to pull out what was left of my hair. There was no resistance as each strand made its way to the tub floor.

My husband woke up and joined me. He was surprised and worried to see me like this. He sat next to me and asked, "Are you okay?" He knew how fond I was of my thick dark hair. It was my crowning glory; something I had always taken pride in.

I asked him if he could help me pull the last of my locks out. He did. I noticed that he shook a little bit as he sat there with me. It must have been traumatic for him too. It was a heavily emotional moment. At the end of this process, there was still some hair left to be shaved off. This is when he put his arm around me and I cried.

We found a clipper to shave the rest. The buzzing noise and bathroom chat woke my parents up and they joined us. Both in shock, they tried to force a smile. My mom looked sympathetic and dad had tears in his eyes. Once Raj had shaved my head, I looked at myself in the mirror and remember saying, "I still look good." We all smiled. It was a smile of acceptance of the new, bald me.

For the next few days, I couldn't help constantly touching my bald head. It was a strange sensation; not entirely unwelcome. It was new. I would even go up to my dad and say, "Touch it. Touch it." He would indulge me each time and remark on how smooth it was.

Anyone with South Asian heritage knows what it's like to be blessed with an ample amount of hair. Those dark, lush, locks cover not only your head, but your body as well. When I wax my arms and legs, I feel 3 kgs lighter. Many of my friends wax their entire bodies. To us, hair removal is a regular part of our lifestyle - just like eating, sleeping, or conversation. If I don't do the monthly yanking of the hair follicles, I can't wear a dress without looking like a hipster man.

Why am I telling you how hairy I am? To showcase the absolute pleasure of not waxing for six to eight months. I finally had time to go grocery shopping, read a book, watch movies, and cook. Losing my bodily hair was one of the best parts of chemotherapy. My skin felt velvety smooth. One quick shower with a loofah scrub and I emerged refreshed, glowing, and silky.

Until I started chemo, I never even gave my nose hair a second thought. A single heavy sigh reminded me that these existed as well, and that they too were bidding me "adieu". If I breathed out too heavily, these tiny strands would zoom out of each nostril at an alarming pace. If I breathed in too deeply, they'd fly the other way, almost clogging my airways.

Badly behaved body hair, I tell you, provided entertainment for days.

When winter rolled around, the hair loss was a little less than fabulous. The frosty air very quickly taught me why we actually have hair all over our bodies. Because my eyelashes fell out, going for a walk on those icy mornings was impossible without tears flooding my cheeks. I couldn't watch television, or read a book, without taking a break every few minutes to wipe my eyes. I often resorted to sticking pieces of tissue below my eyes so that I wouldn't have to go through the constant wiping motions, allowing me to watch my shows in peace.

Breathing felt different. The air felt colder and harsher in my nose and throat. The hairs, which usually act as filters, were no longer there, so I felt the volume of air that came in and out of my nasal passage more intensely than before. There were times when I breathed in tiny fruit flies, unidentified bugs, debris, and anything else that flew around at nose height. I had never appreciated my nose hairs until that point.

When I eventually began to regrow the hair on my scalp, barely visible and stubbly though it was, I massaged castor oil into it as frequently as possible. I wanted to do all I could to encourage healthy hair growth. There were times when I was cooking - boiling pasta or something - when I would lean over the stove and steam my scalp. I was a desperate woman, believing that the steam would open up my pores and help with the absorption of the nourishing oil. Heck, I was pretty sure the amazing nutrients trapped in the steam would help my stubble on its journey to becoming real hair again. The breakdown in proteins and carbohydrates would almost definitely aid in hair growth...

There was no danger of my hair falling in the food, so I saw no harm in playing the odds.

Then there was the constant struggle in shower, a dilemma I faced every time I tried to choose between either body wash or shampoo to use on my head.

SKIN

I was a very sheltered child. My parents, in the fear of spoiling their only child, were strict about everything. Doing make-up or wearing fancy clothes while growing up was a no-no.

Going to a catholic boarding school didn't lift the restrictions either. The school was a lot more particular about 'decorating faces and bodies'. So, throughout my boarding school years, we girls weren't allowed to use makeup. When I eventually left that school and started at a new high school, my mother gave me some (very limited) makeup. At this juncture, I discovered the wondrous nature of glitter, which soon became near-obsession.

While the rest of the world was following hip-hop culture, with loose-fitting, baggy clothes, one very special teenage girl in Nepal was fixated on glitter. I never missed a chance to use it - and use it liberally. My neck, arms, face, legs... You name it, I glitterfied it. I was a 15-year-old in the body of a 7-year-old. I was a magnificent unicorn. I wanted to stay that way and I am not ashamed to confess it. After chemo, with hot flashes and sweats, my entire body glowed with shiny droplets. This wasn't 'normal person' sweat. It wasn't a gym or hot yoga glow. This was cellular. Every tiny cell in my body excreted sweat, making it look like I had flecks of natural glitter all over my body.

I was a glittering embodiment of my teenage self - and I didn't even need to sprinkle products on myself to achieve it.

When I started to properly experience hot flashes at the age of 33, in the middle of winter, what a joy it was! I could suddenly walk around in shorts and tank tops. I was defying the chill and basking in my own glorious warmth.

The magic faded a little when it started happening more frequently; multiple times a day. Each hot flash always started with the feeling of someone trying to tie a knot in my stomach, after which my sweat glands started to move against gravity and rise up. Before long, I was sweating profusely.

Hot flashes, sweats, and chills are common side effects of chemotherapy. For those, like myself, who are on endocrine (hormone) treatment, this is a common phenomenon. Although it has now been over 3 years of experiencing hot flashes, I can tell you, I am still not used to it.

It's hard to put it into words how someone feels when they have hot flashes. Apart from a knot in your stomach, there is a sudden sensation of dizziness and faintness in your head, coupled with surges of emotion. I have had moments where I have been in the midst of an important meeting and I have started to sweat without control. It's often so noticeable that I have been asked by clients if I am okay.

I have found yoga and pranayam (breathing) to be an effective way to keep the hot flashes at bay. I have given up eating or drinking things that make my episodes worse. For as long as I am on medication, I need to manage the hot flash "peaks" when I feel them coming on and make sure they are kept under control.

TASTE & STOMACH

For a foodie, taste is everything: that first bite of a juicy burger, the explosions of spices when you take that first mouthful of Pad Krapow, the crispy bitter freshness of a rocket salad, or the creamy coffee taste of tiramisu. Our tongue does wonders to recognise and satisfy our hunger and passion for food.

One of the saddest experiences for me was the inability to enjoy food for almost a year. It was hard and it hurt me badly. My appetite changed and so did my tastes. I could never accept that I did not like eating, or even the smell or sight of food during this time. At one point, even the smell of water made me gag. YES! Even water has a smell and I couldn't help but hate it for some time.

I was told over and over again how important it was to eat, to recover, and to improve my immune system. So, everything I ate was thick and soupy, almost like it was made in a baby food processor. I found myself having to count to three and quickly swallow, without giving my tastebuds a chance to engage with anything I consumed.

While food was NOT my friend, cravings did happen. Cravings for fancy foods that required a lot of chewing were the worst. Two things would always happen to me when these hit. First, on the third bite, I would always get tired. My body was so weak that, by this point, my jaw had already worked to its capacity. Second, by the time I'd taken a few bites, the taste or smell of the food just wouldn't be appetising anymore.

I found myself stuck within the dilemma of, "How do I get better or stronger if I don't feel like eating?" For that, my friends, I found the perfect solution. If you imagine yourself not having any teeth and not being able to chew food, the best option is to make some kind of a stew. Take the food you're craving - let's say, pasta - and blend the ingredients together into an easily swallowable consistency. I ate a lot of soups (no chunks), smoothies, and Jaulo (the soupier version of Khichadi). With this nifty little trick, by the time I realised I didn't like the taste of food, I was already done with dinner.

Let me share with you how crazy my cravings really were. At one point in my journey, I was in the hospital for five days. The secluded, germ-free facility was as bland in its food offerings as it was in atmosphere. After a few hospital-grade meals, my inner desi woke up. I was aching for some spicy Indian or Nepali food. Unfortunately, there weren't many Indian and Nepali restaurants close by, so I asked my husband to grab me some Katsu curry. I figured it would be an adequate substitute - especially when the craving was so strong.

My husband ran off on the all-important mission to satisfy my cravings. I was so excited that I could finally eat food from the outside world. I thought my body MUST be telling me that I was recovering. After all, only a healthy body would crave something so strongly. I was ecstatic that I still craved spices. Thank the Gods, my family wouldn't need to disown me and my boring palate.

As I opened the box of Katsu curry and rice, my desi happiness hormones were doing a Bollywood dance. But, as the first waft of the meal hit my nose, I found myself slamming the box shut with lightning-fast reflexes. I just couldn't bear the smell. I tried to hide my emotions and squash my gag reflexes for my husband's sake. My body lost the battle and I threw up, feeling dejected and only slightly mortified.

The sedulous person that I am, I wanted to give it another try. My next craving was for pasta. More specifically, I wanted a dish from *Padella*, an amazing restaurant near London bridge, which has always been one of my favourites. Raj ran to my rescue. To our dismay, they didn't offer takeaway options. Always trying his best to find a creative solution, my husband asked them if he could bring a container from home. He explained that his wife was in hospital and craving some Italian deliciousness.

They wouldn't budge. So, I had to settle for some noodles from another spot. Despite the drama, I still couldn't bring myself to eat the meal when it arrived. The scent was just overwhelmingly intense for me. Next, we tried a sandwich and then a burger, with no luck. In the end, I ended up eating half a pizza, which wasn't at all the plan. While I don't mind pizza, it certainly isn't my go-to, unless I'm in Napoli and it's the pizza from *L'Antica Pizzeria da Michele...* My husband feasted on all the rejects. Though perhaps that wasn't quite such a nightmarish task for him after all.

Along with having a terrible taste in my mouth and having zero appetite, chemotherapy also affected my digestive tract quite a bit. I dealt with acid reflux, terrible pain after eating, and constant nausea that, despite the anti nausea medication, just wouldn't go away.

Before I share this next experience, let me tell you a little bit about my mother. An amazing woman, obsessed with cleaning and cleanliness, her table manners are exceptional. Her mannerisms are so formal that she will pardon herself if she has to sneeze at the dinner table, and go to another room. My whole life, I never heard her burp or excrete any form of gas from her nethers. Even in the midst of raging fever or flu, eating politely at the table was of the utmost importance and blowing one's nose was not. If someone dared to blow their nose, sneeze, burp, or fart, my mother would leave the table and not eat anything for the rest of that meal. She would take such behaviour as a personal affront.

Having been raised by such an impeccable example of good manners, when my very close friend asked me how I was doing, I hesitated to give her the details of my intimate intestinal issues. I very uncomfortably shared with her over lunch that I couldn't eat much because my stomach was 'very bad'. She asked me a few questions regarding the details of the 'very bad' situation. I hesitantly said, "I burp and fart a lot. And it isn't normal - it doesn't sound normal." She laughed and said, "Oh stop, you're so funny. We all burp and fart our own way."

Already regretting sharing such an intimate detail, I didn't dare go into any further details. Upon returning home, I told my husband and my parents, who had witnessed the catastrophic sounds of my bodily outlets. My husband looked at me like I'd just told him a terrible joke and said, "Next time would you like me to record it and send it to her? Let's see which category of animal she associates with those sounds."

Towards the end of my treatment, farting and burping around my parents and husband became very comfortable. It was a way for us to figure out how my digestive system was doing that day. To our collective surprise, my mother also had to come to terms with my dysfunctional body and, although she still made THAT face, she managed to give me a pass each time.

Chemotherapy affects gut bacteria and can mess with your digestive system. Other than gas and severe sensitivity to different foods and drinks, heartburn and acid reflux became a common part of my life. I would experience excruciating pain in my chest, especially around the surgery area, thanks to gas-related pain. It happened like clockwork at the same time every day.

I was given various medications and natural remedies, some of which helped. I have shared these later on in the book. Over time, I learned how to deal with my eating habits and incorporated a few things that made life more bearable during those times of pain.

SENSITIVITY AND NAILS

Skin sensitivity was another unexpectedly heavy side effect. I could feel my skin burning under a table lamp. I felt like I had gained some kind of superpower. I could feel the heat from computer screens, the increased body temperature from sitting next to another person, the warmth from room lights, if I was sitting directly underneath them.

Once, I wanted to take some grilled vegetables out of the oven, and the heat burned my skin badly enough that I had to apply aloe vera for three days. The nurses had warned me not to operate the oven and I hadn't listened. It was a painful lesson.

One thing was clear: I would need to learn to let others help me. Stubbornness would get me nowhere. I had a really good excuse to ask for help. If there was any time to be pampered, this was it.

Apart from looking a little worse for wear, I also looked like a 'wannabe goth'. I was warned about light sensitivity on my nails, and it was recommended that I use dark nail polish throughout the treatment. I asked if dark red was an option but was told to choose something darker, like black or dark blue. I couldn't have my nails done at a salon - the risk of infection was too high. So, I spent a lot of my time doing my own nails, which was something I hadn't really done in the past.

Over time, I noticed that the colour of my actual nails changed. They began to look black, blue, and yellow. The shade of a bruised cartoon banana. The dark nail polish, thankfully, helped to hide this frightful sight.

Have you ever thought about what your fingernails are useful for? After my six rounds of chemo, the doctors said it would be a few months before I felt better again. They did, however, forget to tell me that a few of the side effects carry on for some time.

Three months after my last chemo session, my fingers began to shed their nails like a tree shedding its leaves in autumn. The first time I noticed this was when I was trying to pull my jeans up. My nail grazed on the waistband of my jeans and I saw something ping off me and onto the floor. At first, I didn't know what it was. Then I felt a weird pain on my left thumb. A closer look told me that my nail was gone. Ripped off.

A week later, I'd lost a few more. A month later, all ten of my fingers had no nails. To make movement easier and to be able to use my fingers, I tied plasters around my finger tips. I remember not being able to swim in the sea, because the exposed skin right below my nails was burning from the salt water.

Neuropathy is the tingling feeling on the tips of your fingers, hands, toes, or the soles of your feet. A common side effect of Docetaxel, I took pride in not experiencing this particular side effect during my treatment. Almost a year after my chemotherapy, I started to notice that, when I walked too much, I had a tingling sensation on my feet. The only things that helped were soaking them in warm salt water or massaging them with coconut oil.

My father, a humble soul, used to massage my feet every evening, with cold pressed coconut oil. It was almost a part of our daily routine. No matter how tired or sleepy he was, he made sure to massage my feet - even when I protested out of concern for his well being. As a South Asian adult, I had no choice but to respect his decision - respect for your elders is a benchmark of our culture. I'm eternally grateful for this, especially in this instant, the massages really helped ease the pain and helped me sleep better. Even now, the smell of coconut oil reminds me of our father-daughter time.

They say you never know the value of something until it's gone. For me, this was true of my eyelashes, nasal hair, and now also my nails. Many things I had taken for granted, I could not do without my nails. I couldn't hold a pen or a pencil. I couldn't button a shirt. I couldn't zip anything - my purse, my trousers, my jacket. I was unable to put an earring in, and I couldn't scratch my back or my face. I couldn't screw or unscrew a bottle. I couldn't even use my finger-tips to type. All this became an issue months after my treatment was already over.

MEDICINE

You know that movie *Inception*; a dream within a dream within a dream? I was taking medicine to help me with the side effects caused by chemotherapy. Then there were medicines I had to take to help with those medicines, the ones that were helping me with the side effects of the original medicines. It was a convoluted medical mess.

So for example, I had a bad rash on my scalp, which we later found out was due to the anti-nausea medication I was taking. Then, to help me get rid of the rash, I needed additional medicines and ointments.

The injection I was taking to help produce more white blood cells in my body, Filgrastim, was meant to counteract the side effects of Doxatacel, a Chemotherapy drug which reduces your white blood cells. I was already taking a low dose of steroids to combat the negative effects of the chemo, but apparently that just wasn't enough.

Filgrastim stimulates the production of white blood cells, which means your body has to work much faster on this process than it usually does. This has an impact on your system and the injections have side effects. Bad cramps and lower back aches - similar to contractions during pregnancy - were just par for the course. To help with this pain, I was prescribed Co-codamol, which is an incredibly powerful pain medicine. Now, Co-codamol comes with its own side effects, one of which is constipation, along with feeling sick and sleepy. For good measure, we needed to add a laxative to an already long list of medications.

Taking medicines became a necessity. I often felt my life was dependent solely on them. I was impatient and wanted to finish my treatment as quickly as possible. I didn't want to be so heavily reliant on pharmaceuticals. I had to constantly remind myself that my body needed time, my mind needed time, and that everything around me was operating on a time of its own.

This realisation about the fluidity of time is something I had to constantly remind myself of. It's something friends and families should always remind their loved ones of during the treatment process.

Cancer is a lonely disease. It takes up most of a person's time. Half a year to a few years; that's the general time frame for dealing with physical side effects. Emotional side effects can take even longer. Because the treatments and side effects are so different from one person to another, I sometimes find it difficult to explain to people exactly what I was experiencing. The pain in my nail beds or the taste of shampoo in my mouth is entirely subjective - I have no way of knowing if someone else will ever experience this in the same way.

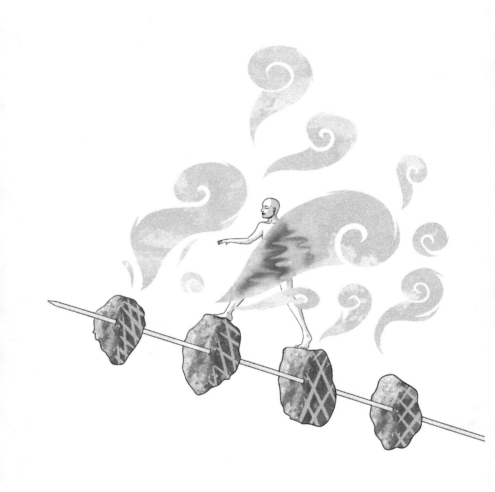

Chapter 5

Sekuwa

Radiotherapy

Sekuwa is meat that is marinated in herbs and spices, then slow-roasted in a natural wood fire. The marinated meat is carefully cubed and skewered, then rotated evenly for a tasty char around the edges and an intensely rich red colour to the meat itself. After I was marinated in a heavy mix of chemo drugs, my breast was tattooed, marked with precious markings and calculations, and I was placed (somewhat unceremoniously) under the GE Discovery RT radiotherapy machine.

Ionising radiation slowly roasts and kills malignant cells, much like the cubes of lamb cooked slowly over an open flame. During my radiotherapy treatment, I was that piece of meat, scorched to (hopeful) perfection.

After six rounds of chemotherapy, it was time to move on to radiotherapy. Where chemo floods your entire body, killing off both the healthy and unhealthy cells, radiotherapy is very localised. It only focuses on the primarily cancerous area.

Not everyone goes through radiotherapy. It was not a unanimous vote for the treatment on my medical team - I was right on the cusp of it being a requirement. After some to and fro, the decision was left to me. I was provided with the potential odds for success along with all the information needed to mull it over on my own.

Lacking the knowledge of a medical professional, I did what anyone would do. I read a lot. I thought even more. And I took the time to speak to others who had opted to go through with radiotherapy treatment on their respective journeys. It was a big decision to make; definitely not one to be taken lightly. I needed to take some time to weigh up my options.

This process reminded me that I truly am blessed with some amazing people in my life. My aunt introduced me to some of her friends in London. One of these wonderful women had been at her mother's side during her breast cancer journey, and had an understanding of what I might be going through. They were good friends with a fantastic oncologist in India, and they made an introduction. This doctor not only took the time to look at my reports but was instrumental in giving me advice at various points during the treatment process. He helped me make the decision to proceed with radiotherapy. I remember him saying, "You've gone through worse, so you have nothing to fear." And he was right.

A dose of 40.05 Gray over 15 treatments was prescribed for my right chest wall. Apparently, that was the lowest dosage I could get in this situation. I'm not sure whether I should have been grateful for this at all. My radiotherapy was scheduled to start in January 2017. Just before Christmas, they called me in to take measurements. Measurements for radiotherapy; the concept made no sense to me at all.

I walked into an uncomfortably cold room with a swanky looking GE machine. I was asked to take my clothes off and lay down on a frosty metal bed, with my right arm above my head. My head, legs, and back were adjusted, and then began the numbers game. Precise measurements were taken of the angle of my foot, leg, arm, and the tilt of my head. I wasn't sure if this was for radiotherapy or if I was going to be included in the wax display at Madame Tussauds.

Two nurses kept an eye on me, both of whom insisted I not move at all. I wasn't even sure if I was allowed to take a deep breath. I was scared my body would move and they would have to take the measurements again. Permanent dots were tattooed on me - one in the centre of my breast, one on the left side and one on the right. Three tiny medical tattoos to add to my other, more rebellious collection. A total of five tattoos - what a wild child! The markings would ensure that every time I came for radiation, it would be targeted at exactly the right place.

Whenever I went into the radiation room, it took the professionals about half an hour just to set me up. They would ask me to slide up or down, then move me in a way that felt like I was a piece of meat, crassly displayed on a slab of ice at the supermarket. My back muscles were adjusted. My legs were either moved apart or pushed together. While it took forever to set me up, the actual radiation only took about 10 minutes. Honestly, it took me longer to undress, put on the gown, and get dressed again than it did to sit still for the treatment.

Once the bed was lowered into position, the nurses would cover me up a bit because I couldn't control my shivering. The cold metal wasn't pleasant but the room needed to be kept cool to protect the radiotherapy machine from overheating. As soon as my body was properly adjusted, I was dragged into the tunnel. Sometimes, I closed my eyes. Other times, I didn't. Claustrophobia wasn't a problem for me. I found solace in being alone and enclosed - I was almost comforted by the machines.

For a while, the noise, the smell of the machine, and the super cold room became a part of my life. For 15 days, this was simply a part of my day. It became totally automatic - a habit. I woke up on the 16th day and got ready for my next session, not realising that they were all done.

The side effects of the radiotherapy are not instant. The delayed side effects can be short term or long term. Some of the side effects continue for a long time after the treatment is over. After chemotherapy, radiotherapy was a walk in the park for me.

Where the radiotherapy was targeted, my skin was always hot and burning, dry and itchy. The burn is quite similar to a sunburn, they told me. My South Asian skin had always protected me from sunburn, so I had no real reference points for this. Google told me what I needed to know, in this case. I used organic aloe vera gel and chemical-free cream to help with the burn. What helped the most was popping these lotions and potions in the fridge before using them. Sweet, soothing relief!

I was told to drink around 4-5 litres of water a day. At first, I thought that was physically impossible. I was tired - exhausted, really - and even drinking water was a tiresome task. When they tell you to drink copious amounts of liquid, you have to find alternatives to just plain water.

I started having a lot of interesting drinks, like homemade ginger ale (refer to my recipe) and mint and cucumber-infused water. I also really got into homemade lemonade - Indian style, both sweet and salty - it's weird at first but it quickly becomes a taste you get used to. The combination of sweet and salty is something people who have grown up in South Asia are used to. This could either be because it's a prevalent part of the cuisine, or because at some point you've been dehydrated enough to make your own electrolyte solution with salt, sugar, and water (too much street food has its downsides). A dash of lemon in that particular electrolyte solution is a serious upgrade.

During and after radiotherapy, I drank a ton of fruit juices and smoothies. Even though it was January and the brisk cold of winter was still heavy in the air, I wanted cold drinks. If I was out and about during the day, I had to refuel every hour because I got tired really easily. I couldn't eat with any regularity or gusto since my appetite hadn't returned yet. The best way to refuel was to fill up on fresh juice and drinks.

Having a cold drink not only meant that I could cool my body from the inside but that I could use the frosty glass as an ice pack. I balanced those glasses on my burning breast every chance I got. It's a great help when you're at home and lounging in your own space. Heck, I occasionally did it when I was outside of the house too. Frankly, there's no shame in making yourself feel better at times like these - there's a way to cool yourself off more or less discreetly. If you're comfy and not being particularly obscene about it, who cares?

I was always tired. "Extreme tiredness" is what the good folks in the medical community call it. It's the most honest term I've ever heard. I was too tired to walk up a flight of stairs, too tired to walk from my bedroom to the toilet. London apartments are tiny, so everything is pretty close together. At the time, just looking at the bathroom door made me tired because I knew the short walk would totally tucker me out.

I was like a newly born baby who needs to be fed every three hours. I needed fluids what seemed like all the time. I now totally understand how Popeye feels after his special dose of spinach. With each "refuel", the rush of energy was unreal. I felt alive, awake, full of energy. I felt like I could conquer Everest, take over the world, walk up the next flight of stairs…

It's different for everyone, though. The treatment experience.

I know of someone who's experience was the complete opposite of mine. Her radiotherapy side effects were much worse than those she dealt with during chemotherapy. Because the dose of chemo was minimal in her case, so were the side effects. Her radiotherapy dose was higher than mine, and her treatment period was longer. She told me that her skin was so badly burnt that it started to peel off. The pain was so unbearable that she had to take medication for it. It also made her tired, flat, and unable to do any chores or go to work. She remained almost totally functional during chemo - business as usual. Her appetite changed and she just didn't have the urge to eat. Her emotional health took a serious knock due to the constant fatigue and her lack of interest in anything.

We all suffer differently.

If chemo made people perceive me as a homeless person, then radiotherapy made me an old woman. During radiotherapy, I aged even more. I was the only 33-year-old, sitting in the waiting room surrounded by 70-80-year-olds. I even started having "old people conversations" with them.

I became good friends with a gentleman who was 82 and was travelling 7 hours just to get to the hospital and back. He used to be a telephone engineer. Together, we bitched about how the mobile phone had changed everyone's life, and how telephone engineers were out of jobs. With another woman, I discussed, in-depth, the side effects of her menopause and my side effects from the medication - hot flashes and sweats. How they were during winter and how terrible the mood swings were.

Most conversations started with 'when I was younger'. This was a reminder that disease knows no age, colour, or gender barriers. It affected us all the same. The best part of all of this was that my husband joined us in all these conversations. I'm sure he enjoyed them as much as I did. These were the best times we spent in the hospital's waiting room.

Months after the treatment ended, some side effects continued to creep up on me. Occasional pain around the chest area, random sharp pricking pain at any given moment, and hardening of the muscle around the target area - these were just a few of them. I also used to feel my ribs ache at times. This can even happen years down the line.

I started to have capsular contracture (a response of the body's immune system to foreign materials) around my right implant and breast area. The pain was excruciating and the only cure was replacement surgery, which I eventually underwent a year later.

As my physical side effects began to subside, it was the psychological side effects I was left to deal with.

CURRY

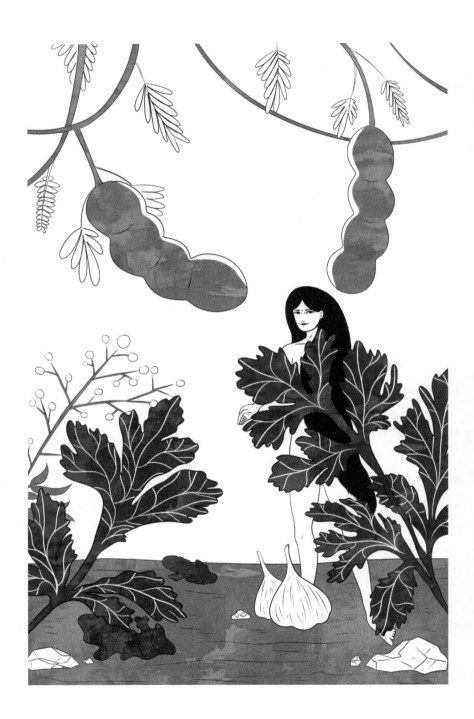

Herbs and Spices

Flavour, Comfort, Healing

In the summer of 2000, at the age of 17, I decided I wanted to pierce my nose. This isn't particularly uncommon in my culture. Young girls pierce their noses as a symbol of purity (don't get me started on the explanation or the reasoning behind some cultural beliefs). Although one of the first gifts I received as a baby was a gold and diamond nose ring, my family isn't overly religious, so the piercing issue wasn't a pressure point. Not until I hit my teens and began exploring a new-found love of tattoos and piercings.

My mother discouraged me from the piercing, since it was summer and the chances of infection were a little higher than normal. Backed by courage that I feared would waiver if I waited, I went ahead and got it pierced anyway. A few days later, my nose was swollen and red, fully infected.

My mother almost left me to deal with my misery alone, since I hadn't listened to her. Aching for sympathy, I turned to my maternal grandmother, Ma. Spending the weekend with her turned out to be the right choice. Her Ayurvedic knowledge is boundless. To heal my Rudolph-like nose, she made a paste of turmeric and mustard oil that needed to be applied to the offending area several times a day. Three days later, my nose was completely yellow from the turmeric but the infection was almost gone.

I give Ma all the credit for my appreciation of spices and naturopathy. She taught me that you can brush your teeth with turmeric and mustard oil for whitening long before it became a viral YouTube trend. She gave me a spoonful of dried ginger soaked in honey when I had a sore throat. She cooked up a stew made with *Jwano* (or Carom) seed, potatoes and tomatoes to eat with rice when I had a bad stomach ache. She also showed me that you can pack black pepper, cloves, and Sichuan peppers in tiny cloth pouches that can be stored in cupboards to keep termites and worms at bay.

Ma taught me that spices are not only a part of the kitchen, they're a part of life.

After cancer, I developed an even deeper interest in the healing properties of spices. I'm not saying that they are an alternative to pharmaceutical drugs, but they certainly helped me through some of the toughest parts of my treatment cycle.

Ayurvedic knowledge has been around for over 5000 years. Ayurveda focuses on the overall well-being of a person. This includes the mind, soul, and physical body. According to Ayurveda, the five elements of nature - space, air, fire, water, and earth - are present in our bodies in three categories (*doshas*). *Vatta* is air and space, *Pitta* is fire and water, and *Kapha is* earth and water.

Imbalance in any of the five elements results in illness or other manifestations of ill health in the physical body. Therapies are based on complex herbal compounds, metals, and minerals, most of which are available to us in nature.

In India, and some parts of the world, Ayurvedic medicines still hold a sacred place in people's lives. Some believe it to be a curative option, while others view it as preventive. Either way, it is an important part of most Asians' lives, including mine.

My mother often talks about how, as a baby, I often bled from my anus. (After discussing my smashed breasts and gastric issues, I'm not particularly intimidated by these kinds of stories anymore. Can you tell?) I was taken to see all the best pediatricians in the country, none of whom were able to heal my unknown condition. Eventually, someone recommended a *Baidhya* (Ayurvedic doctor) who was well-known in the country. Having had no luck with Western medicine, my parents decided it was worth a try. The *Baidhya* examined me and gave my parents a few herbal pouches with some carefully written instructions attached. A few days later, I was okay.

Since then, until the *Baidhya* passed away, I used to see him regularly.

In the UK, Ayurveda or Ayurvedic treatment is considered a complementary and alternative medicine (CAM). With very little research or medical evidence to support claims of healing, there are many scientists and medical professionals that do not recognise its use as a legitimate medicine. Yet, there are many who think otherwise. Personally, during my cancer treatment, I only used some herbs and spices to help me with the side effects. Now, however, I follow a holistic lifestyle and believe in Ayurvedic healing as a preventive measure.

I am not a total naturalist. I do still believe in pharmaceutical medicines and their life-altering abilities.

When taking antibiotics becomes a common occurrence, one builds resilience towards it. During my treatment I was taking antibiotics after almost every session of chemo, roughly five times in six months. Paracetamol and ibuprofen seemed insufficient, and I had to switch to a stronger prescription of codeine for pain relief. The same goes for many other medicines. We certainly do need them, but I slowly learned to cope with some side effects just by using the natural herbs and spices available in my kitchen cabinet.

My nausea drastically reduced when I sucked on ginger. So I regularly had ginger drinks, home-made of course. My gas and stomach problems began to subside when I chose to eat more mint, *Jwano* (*ajwain*), and aloe vera, in every meal.

We live in fortunate times where our world has become smaller. I live in London but I know that in every major city, supermarkets now carry spices from all over the globe. Wars are no longer fought over trade and spices. Spices are no longer more expensive than gold, diamonds, or silver.

We've come a long way since Christopher Columbus and the Dutch East India Trading Company. Spices are not only for the rich and privileged few. Nepali food, which is similar to Indian food, uses less spices. So, really, it's a blander version of a familiar favourite.

Nepal, with its topography could not grow many spices. Historically, the country also couldn't afford to buy spices from India - though that's not the case today. However, the spices that are grown locally - Sichuan peppercorns, green cardamom, and nutmeg - can be found abundantly in Nepali food.

Spices give food, taste, texture and aroma. Some spices are versatile and can be used in many different forms. For example, cilantro (coriander) can be consumed as a fresh leafy herb, or the dried seeds can be used as a spice (powdered or whole). The fresh roots, when finely chopped, are great too.

Some spices are hot and have a really strong kick and, when used in minimal amounts, will not only improve the taste of food, but also help your body. Then again, not all spices bring the burn and are more aromatic - adding subtle nuances of flavour and colour.

Understanding spices and what they can do for you during your treatment is important. Only you understand how your body reacts, what it craves, and what it doesn't. Tastes and flavours vary and so do your choices. It's a little less overwhelming if you spend some time getting to know about the use of these spices in both cooking and healing processes.

I always carry a small box filled with cloves, green cardamom, and cinnamon sticks cut into small pieces. You will find similar boxes in the purses of my mum, grandmother, and aunt. In fact, you'll probably find these boxes in most Nepali women's purses. I pop a small amount into my mouth as a breath freshener or to soothe my stomach after a heavy meal. Clove is a powerful remedy for gum and toothache while cardamom and cinnamon help aid digestion and mask strong food aromas. This magical little combo is great for coffee drinkers or onion and garlic lovers. I fall into the latter category myself.

Here are some of the spices used on the Indian/ Nepali subcontinent. They might be useful for some of the recipes that I share later on.

I would like to quickly touch on how these spices helped me in the process of my treatment and recovery, and what benefits they have.

ASAFOETIDA | *HING*

I can never pronounce this one. Asafoetida gets its name from Latin, where "foetida" means "stinky". This distant cousin of celery and onion shares a similar pungent taste and smell. Once cooked, though, it mellows down a lot. If you think you've never heard of this or eaten it, you're probably wrong. If you've been to an Indian restaurant, you've wolfed it down without even knowing it.

Asafoetida is one of the main ingredients in Pappads or, as the rest of the world so lovingly calls them, papadums. It is said to be native to the Iran/ Afghanistan area, so it was most likely brought to the Indian sub-continent by the Persians.

Benefits:

Asafoetida is said to contain polyphenols, which are powerful antioxidants found in green tea and dark chocolate. When cooking lentils or especially beans in India and Nepal, Asafoetida is a must. It helps reduce the production of gas when too many beans are guzzled. Go on, you probably know the rhyme... They're good for the heart!

Asafoetida makes it easier for vegetarians and vegans to consume lentils and beans regularly, without the embarrassing digestive jamboree.

Asafoetida was used in the 1918 influenza pandemic to stave off infection. People walked around with small pouches of Asafoetida tied around their necks. It was also sanctioned by the US Pharmacopeia, the organisation that set standards for medicine at the time. Many years later, when the swine flu broke out, researchers in Egypt and Taiwan discovered that Asafoetida killed the swine flu virus more effectively than Amantadine, an antiviral drug used to control the disease.

How to use it:

It can be used in daals, lentils, while cooking any kind of beans, curries, and meats. The main use of Asafoetida in the Middle East is to tenderise meat. As bad as it smells in its powder form, when added to food, you won't notice the smell or taste anymore.

It should be added to dishes at the beginning of the cooking process, when the oil warms up. This helps mellow the smell and flavour of the spice. Sometimes, it is also added towards the end when tempering a dish is required. If you are making anything curry based (pie, samosa, *chaat*) you can always add *hing*.

To get the most of its health benefits, you can even add it to soups and stews. The aroma and taste will be completely masked but the health benefits are all there.

BISHOPS WEED SEEDS | *JWANO* | *AJWAIN*

Jwano seeds are incredibly nutritious, rich in fiber, vitamins and minerals and known for its antioxidant properties. They have been used in Ayurvedic medicines for a long time.

In Indian cuisine, *Jwano* seeds are tempered in ghee or oil when preparing a dish. This is often the point at which cumin seeds are toasted off as well. In Nepali cuisine, you won't see these two spices together. In other Asian countries, they're considered a perfectly balanced pair.

In Nepal we use *Jwano* solely to prepare a thin, almost translucent soup to eat with rice. I've included this recipe a little later on in this book.

Benefits:

Jwano contains thymol and carvacrol, both of which are well-known for their antibacterial and antifungal properties. It also helps to balance the pH balance in the gut, stopping the growth of candida. This is why it's so widely used to help treat stomach aches in South Asia.

This spice is great for relieving pain caused by ulcers and gas-related indigestion in the upper stomach. These are the types of issues often caused by chronic constipation.

When applied as a paste on a child's chest, *Jwano* helps to make breathing easier and gets rid of persistent coughing.

If you don't cook Indian food often, or at all, you can always add Jwano seeds to bread or wraps, for a bit of variation in flavour. The seeds are an interesting addition to soups or meat and vegetables dishes, provided you remember to toast them off first. A little bit of heat brings out its almost thyme-like aroma.

How to use it:

As amazing as *jwano* can be in curries, you can use this humble seed in almost everything. It goes very well with bread, either sprinkled on top or mixed through the dough. It's particularly tasty when included in homemade flatbreads and pita.

When toasted, it can be sprinkled on top of salads and hummus, or any savoury dips. It also makes a wicked stew for those who have cold and chesty coughs, and aids with the production of breast milk in pregnant/ breastfeeding mothers.

CARDAMOM | *ELAICHI*

Did you know that cardamom is the world's third most expensive spice after vanilla and saffron? I didn't. An essential ingredient in garam masala, it's what makes a good curry "sing". A small pinch of this spice goes a long way. If you're heavy handed, you might end up with more bitterness than you can handle.

The smell of cardamom brings back memories of my grandmother whipping up some sweet delight, while I waited with baited breath to see what she'd come up with. Although it's also used in savory food, adding cardamom to a dessert just makes it a thousand times better. With it's heady, almost perfumey aroma, it's no wonder this spice is so popular.

The seeds, which is what cardamom is all about, are nestled inside green or black pods. Grown in Nepal, black cardamom is known to be the best. The green pods, on the other hand, are found in India and some South Asian countries.

Benefits:

Cardamon was once chewed by the Romans as an alternative for brushing their teeth.It keeps gingivitis at bay and promotes healthy teeth and gums. It is also used by many to help promote a healthy gut. Cardamom has anti- inflammatory and antispasmodic properties, helping to decrease stomach muscle spasms.

In Ayurvedic treatment, cardamom is also used to combat sinus problems, asthma, or general breathing issues.

How to use it:

During my treatment, I often chewed on cardamom when that soapy taste lingered in my mouth. If it's strong enough to combat garlic breath, it's strong enough to get rid of that post-chemo assault on the taste buds.

Although I am a (mostly) rice-eating person, there were points during my treatment when the smell of rice just wasn't appealing. My mum used to add two to three cardamom pods to the pot while boiling the rice. It helped to mask the stodgy, glutinous smell of the steam and helped to restore my appetite.

I also used to steep cinnamon, clove, and cardamom powder in warm water as a soothing drink. The taste of real Indian masala chai - is there anything better? It gave me a break from the seemingly never-ending stream of tea. A spoonful of honey transformed it into a real moreish delight - something healthy to curb the occasional craving for something sweet.

Plain yogurt can quickly and easily be jazzed up with some honey and cardamom powder. Cardamom also goes very well with apple pie and rice pudding. It's unbelievably versatile.

CINNAMON | *DAALCHINI*

My love for this spice developed only recently, after I discovered cinnamon buns and cinnamon toast crunch. The sweet smell and delicate taste is something I crave even now.

There are two types of cinnamon. Chinese Cinnamon or Chinese Cassia (Cinnamomum Cassia), is commonly used in baked goods, desserts, and cereals. The other, which is the "true" cinnamon or Ceylon cinnamon (Cinnamomum Verum), is produced mostly in Sri-lanka. The latter option is what you should look for. This is the one that has the true flavour and all the health benefits.

In the UK, it's easy to tell the difference - read the label. You can also tell the difference between the two by looking at them. Cassia is a darker reddish brown whereas true cinnamon is light brown in colour. Also take note of the shape of the sticks. True cinnamon comes in layers within a tube, flaky and thin. Cassia, on the other hand, has distinctive double scrolls in thicker pieces. It is very important to use the right cinnamon. Although there are no serious disadvantages to consuming cassia, there are no benefits either.

Benefits:

Cinnamon reduces blood sugar levels, cutting the risk of heart disease by a whole lot. It's also loaded with antioxidants, therefore making it a superfood.

How to use it:

Cinnamon is commonly used in desserts in the Western world, but its use goes beyond just sweets. It is used to flavour sweet and savory dishes in Asian, South Aisian, Chinese, Latin American, and African cuisine.

Because I needed to stay hydrated during my radiotherapy, a few cinnamon sticks steeped in a tea pot filled with boiling water was something I used to sip on all day. The comforting aroma and slight sweetness makes it some much more enjoyable to drink than plain water. Cinnamon infused water is now a favourite drink that my mum and I enjoy while watching television - hot during winter and cold during summer.

Lassi, a yogurt based drink very popular in India, and the smoothies that I make at home, will always have a pinch of cinnamon. Mango-based lassis and smoothies, in particular, benefit from a sprinkling of this fabulous spice.

A few sticks of cinnamon added to a pot of boiling rice, transforms a bland side into something completely different. In fact, without cinnamon, Pilau rice just wouldn't taste right at all.

If you have ever made apple sauce at home, you will know that cinnamon is essential while you're cooking down the fruit. When chewing fruit - like apples or pears - was difficult for me during chemotherapy, I used to bake those fruits with some cinnamon and eat them as snacks.

Although the smell and taste of eggs didn't quite tickle my fancy during chemo, I can really enjoy a luscious bread pudding or stack of French toast now. When those items are on the menu, it's the perfect chance for cinnamon to shine.

CLOVE | *LUWANG*

Growing up, dental problems were something I was all too familiar with. Mamu often dabbed a bit of clove oil on a piece of cotton and would press it gently against the offending tooth. The less enjoyable option was to bite ferociously into a few whole cloves to release the oil onto the affected area. To this day, I can't help but associate cloves with dental pain.

If you have ever hastily bitten into a clove, you might be familiar with the instant numbness it causes. Eugenol, the oil present in clove bud, is great for tooth or gum problems. It's another spice that's great for combatting bad breath. Originally, from Indonesia, these dried flower buds are now grown in many countries.

Cloves have been used in medicinal applications for centuries. In fact, humans used cloves in medicine long before they made their way to the kitchen. When I was younger, my mother would dab a bit of clove oil on some cotton wool and place it directly on my gum to battle an aching tooth.

Cloves are used in many Asian cuisines. It's yet another one of the components that make a great garam masala. South Asian and European cuisines, especially, tend to add this somewhat "Christmassy" spice to pies and hot drinks.

Benefits:

Nausea is one of the most common side effects associated with chemotherapy. The drugs also affect the inner lining of the stomach, resulting in gas, abdominal pain, bloating, diarrhea, or constipation. Clove is the perfect natural remedy for all of those gastric ailments.

How to use it:

Apart from sucking or chewing on a single clove in its simplest state, I used it in a whole lot of my cooking. For almost instant relief from nausea, I would make a warm or cold drink with cloves, cinnamon, and cardamom, either with milk or without.

If you are making soups or stews, you can always use 2-3 cloves to add flavour and reap the medicinal benefits. Just be sure to take those them out before blending the soup or dishing up the stew.

Fishing cloves out of a pot of food can be a little frustrating. To make your life easier, stud a few cloves in a small whole onion before chucking it in the pot. When the dish is done, just yank out the onion and you'll have all of the flavour with none of the fuss.

CORIANDER | *DHANIYA*

Coriander is the proverbial "icing on the cake" to any desi dish. It enhances flavours, adds brightness, and ties the dish together.

Coriander leaves, also known as cilantro, are a fairly pungent herb used in many Asian and Latin American dishes. The seeds, on the other hand, are used as an earthy spice either whole or as a powder. In Nepali and Indian cooking, coriander powder is often paired with cumin powder. The seeds are widely used in savory and sweet dishes, not only in Indian cooking, but also in Malaysia, Egypt, Morocco, and Latin American cuisines.

There are two main types of coriander. One is European and the other Indian. The tan-coloured European seeds are bigger than the yellow-ish Indian ones. Both are equally flavourful and used in the same applications. European ones are slightly more flowery and a bit closer to the flavours of celery, whereas Indian coriander seeds are more zesty and lemony.

Benefits:

Apart from imparting amazing flavour to your food, coriander also helps soothe your stomach. Much like asafoetida, adding coriander to beans can make them less heavy on the stomach.

During my treatment, the flavour profile of coriander helped my appetite. This made it a great addition to almost any dishes I cooked during that time. It also helped ease my stomach pain and indigestion. It also lowers your blood sugar levels and while this may not have been an issue for me, it's still a health perk.

How to use it:

The best way to coriander is to buy the seeds whole and grind them just before cooking. It's also fine to use them whole. The seeds remain fresh and the oils intact until they are added to a dish. This isn't a hard and fast rule, though. If you're into convenience, you can buy powdered coriander seeds in small packets like I do.

If you're adding cumin powder to a savoury dish, it's probably a good idea to add coriander too. These two spices are the best of friends. It's great in any curry and makes a fantastic rub for meat. I also add it to soups.

Honestly, coriander often helps me hide my mistakes when cooking. If you've added too much turmeric or cinnamon, bang some coriander in. If you've overdone it with the lemon or chillies, a sprinkling of coriander will save the day.

CUMIN SEEDS | *JEERA*

You can use cumin in almost anything. Very common in Middle Eastern and Indian food, cumin seeds can be used in powder form or left whole. Cumin works well in stews, BBQ rubs, burger patties, salad dressings, or Chinese noodles. Some Italian dishes use cumin too. Try adding it to a bolognese sauce for a surprisingly tasty fusion dish.

Not to be confused with black cumin, Jeera looks a lot like caraway. The seeds - if munched on their own - are quite pungent and bitter. When added sparingly to dishes, cumin adds a more pleasing aroma.

In Nepali food, just like in Indian food, we use cumin seeds and cumin powder in the same dish. It is used to temper daal. We add cumin seeds at the beginning of the cooking process to release all of those beautiful oils. We tend to add the powder during the rest of the cooking process to impart even more flavour.

Benefits:

Cumin is a great source of iron. It's also rich in vitamins A and C, making it the perfect antioxidant that'll keep your blood sugar levels in check.

Adding cumin to your food improves cholesterol, decreases high blood pressure, and aids with digestion. In homeopathy, cumin is given to people who struggle with diabetes. My grandfather used to drink cumin soaked overnight in water when he was diagnosed with diabetes. He never took any medicines, but rather included this routine and other healthy eating habits for the rest of his life. His diabetes never escalated.

How to use it:

Eating rice is a huge part of my culture. If you love rice as much as I do, you'll relish the opportunity to do something different with your rice every now and then. Jeera rice is one of my absolute favourites. During chemo, when plain rice became too boring, jeera rice was a delicious side dish I could eat as a meal on its own.

I learnt how to make jeera rice when I lived in India. I never thought I'd feel the need to jazz up my rice. Rice was rice. The best way to have it was boiled and that was it. My conservative mindset changed when our cook in India made jeera rice for guests one day. It's so easy to make it but the flavour is next level stuff. Once the rice is cooked, toast some cumin seeds in a dry pan until they begin to darken slightly and you can smell those fragrant oils. One tablespoon of cumin seeds per cup of rice should do. Mix it all together, with a spoonful or two of ghee for a more luxurious mouthfeel.

Have you ever had a salty lassi? Next time you do, try adding some crushed, roasted cumin to it. When you take a sip, you'll still be able to bite into the seeds. When I needed to drink ridiculous amounts of liquid, homemade savory lassis were a thirst-quenching staple. It also helped that both the yogurt and cumin were good for my stomach.

Cumin can also be added to roast potatoes, if you want to impress your guests with something a little different. Add seeds to the potatoes before you roast them, along with some good quality olive oil and a sprinkling of coarse sea salt. If you'd prefer to use powder, remember to do so when the potatoes come out of the oven. The powder burns more easily, so you want to avoid that at all costs.

Rubbing cumin onto any type of meat is an extremely satisfying part of the cooking process. It works well with lamb, chicken, beef, and pork. Cumin adds a slightly smokey flavour to the meat, and helps achieve a more intense char.

If you're on a strict diet, cumin can make plain foods more appealing. My mum often added cumin powder to boiled vegetables to make them more palatable. Cumin can make stronger smelling veggies, like broccoli and cauliflower, taste a little "friendlier" too.

FENNEL | *SAUNF*

Ever wondered why some Indian restaurants offer fennel or candied fennel at the end of a meal? It helps freshen your breath after onion, garlic, and heavily spiced meals while aiding in digestion.

The flavour profile is a little divisive. You either love it or you hate it. It has a slight aniseedy tang to it - reminding most people of licorice. If the flavour is up your alley, you'll be pleased by the many uses of the seeds, bulb, and leaves.

The ancient Romans, Greeks, and Indian Ayurvedas used fennel to treat a variety of digestive problems. It's mild enough to use for infants, which means it's generally quite safe for the most sensitive people.

An age old remedy in the West is drinking warm milk infused with fennel. This helps with digestive problems or stomach cramps. In India, I often found fennel in my tea when someone offered me a cup (without milk). I must say, I've been hooked on it ever since. It's fairly normal to find Indian people chewing on fennel seeds to prevent constipation, ease stomach aches, and solve a multitude of digestive issues.

Fennel is also great for treating a cough or sore throat. Try adding a few fennel seeds to black tea. It'll tone down the smell, ease up the flavour, and create a soothing drink that is better than any cough syrup.

In South Asia, *fennel leaf saunf ko saag* is a very common vegetable dish. The bulb is something I only encountered once I came to the UK. I noticed it raw in salads or in soups and stews. Just one cup of fennel bulb contains 2.7 - 2.9 grams of fiber, which automatically does wonders for constipation. The bulb is also high in potassium, vitamin C, and folate which makes it a great addition to any healthy, balanced diet.

Just like dill, fennel is also good with fish, like salmon, seeds are used in a lot of Rye breads and some sausages.

Benefits:

During my treatment process, there were times the smell of fennel repelled me, then there were times I didn't mind it at all. On days where the fennel was bearable, I noticed how helpful it was in combatting the side effects of several medications. Fennel seeds helped with that nasty flavour I had in my mouth and also helped to keep my guts feeling less gassy and sore.

How to use it:

When I was going through chemo, I ate a lot of *saunf saag.* "Saag" is basically any leafy green cooked with garlic and some spices. Nepali saags are made by stir frying the greens in hot oil with garlic and adding salt. Once the leaves wilt, they are taken off the heat and served.

Drinking fennel water, after allowing the seeds to soak overnight, was a great alternative to plain water during radiotherapy. The stronger I made it, the more I felt like I was drinking Pastis (apéritif from France) or Raki (Turkish alcohol). Both of these drinks are made with anise but taste similar. This was my way of feeling like I was still a part of the game.

The use of fennel outside of my treatment has now become a regular part of my life. I make tea, use fennel bulbs in salads, and regularly snack on candied fennel which I got from India.

FENUGREEK SEEDS | *METHI SEEDS*

I have a love-hate relationship with Methi. The leaves of the fenugreek plant are enjoyed as saag (vegetables) and the seeds are used for their massively powerful nutritional value. The seeds have been used in Ayurveda and Chinese medicine for centuries.

If you can increase the consumption of fenugreek during cancer treatment, it will only help. There are many ways you can do it. It can be sprinkled into bread crumbs as a base when you want to fry meat. It can easily be added to any curry at the beginning of the cooking process. A small pinch of it goes well with any dipping sauce; it almost tastes like mustard.

My love for fenugreek is a little limited. I love the *saag* - give me any greens and I am sold. Nepalis have a *saag* for every season. Fenugreek greens taste nothing like the seeds. Brown and hard as a rock, you don't want to try them raw. If you do manage to bite into it, you'll struggle with the bitterness. Once soaked or tempered with hot oil, the seeds are only slightly bitter with an almost maple or oak-like flavour. Woody but not sweet.

As a child I remember my mother soaking and making a paste of fenugreek, which she applied to her hair to promote growth. Breastfeeding mothers were advised to eat more fenugreek because it helped produce more breast milk. In fact, it is one of the key ingredients in *Sutkeri ko Masala,* a dietary supplement given to nursing and postnatal mothers. In Ayurvedic medicine, fenugreek is used to treat or reduce diabetes, weight loss, kidney stones, and infections.

My fondness doesn't extend to fenugreek seeds. If you've cooked with them, you'll know that the pungent smell lingers in the house for days. It's almost impossible to get rid of. I use this spice very rarely. There are only a few things I will add it to.

My relationship with fenugreek seeds took a nasty turn when I signed up for a detox programme a while back. As part of my daily routine, I had to drink fenugreek water, made by soaking the seeds overnight in some purified water. The taste was totally bearable, the issue was what came afterwards. My sweat and urine smelled like fenugreek - maybe even worse. Fenugreek facilitates the secretion of sweat, helping to get rid of toxins from the body.

I did not use fenugreek very much during my treatment, mainly because its strong odour was something I couldn't cope with. When my mom made *jaulo* (recipe provided later on) she added fenugreek, though the taste and smell wasn't quite so strong. I tried to replicate the dish when mother was not around. I took a "more is more" approach, adding a tablespoon of fenugreek to a one-person portion of *jaulo*. The taste was so overpowering that I had to fish each seed out. Luckily, it's easy to spot them since they turn dark brown once added to hot oil. From then on, I couldn't stomach the taste or smell of fenugreek.

Luckily, my intense dislike for fenugreek did eventually pass. Although it still isn't my favourite, I do sometimes cook with it.

How to use it:

Methi seeds can be used in many cooking applications. Almost all Nepali cooking can include a sprinkling of this spice. Similar to *hing* and turmeric, *methi* seeds must be added at the beginning of the cooking process, and can be consumed once they are dark brown/almost black. Even then, when you chew it, you might think you have bitten into a stone.

Other than that we regularly soak *methi* seeds overnight, sprout them for a few days and add them to salads, or make a salad based on the seeds themselves.

GARLIC | LASOON | LASAN

Who doesn't like garlic? I've heard Europeans, Indians, Chinese, Thais, and so many others say, "We can't do without garlic." It's an absolute staple.

To me, garlic is the soul of any hearty, homely, savoury dish. Cooked, raw, dry, powdered... I use it without fail in almost everything I make. We South Asians say we can't cook without garlic and onions, which is true. Everything - and I mean absolutely EVERYTHING - with exception of desserts, has garlic in it.

I've heard somewhere that garlic and onion are perhaps the oldest cultivated crops in the world. Archeological evidence suggests that our forefathers planted these alliums as early as 5000 - 7000 years ago. They were found in the tombs of the Egyptian pharaohs.

Ayurveda suggests that we start the day with a clove of garlic instead of coffee. It's supposed to keep you awake and energised all day. I know many people who swallow cloves of garlic just like they would swallow pills. Wash them down with a glass of water - vampires be damned!

Who cares about garlic breath when you can reap so many benefits? Garlic bread, garlic butter, garlic sauce... How can you worry about your breath when it's so darn tasty?

There is a fix for this, of course. Pop some fennel and cloves in your purse and you'll keep the dragon breath at bay, like I do!

Benefits:

Garlic contains allicin, a compound which converts to organosulfurs. This is where the pungent, zingy taste and smell comes from. The organosulfur in garlic is what minimises the oxidation and inflammation processes in our bodies, making it a powerful antioxidant. It is said to be an ancient remedy for anti-aging and keeping infections at bay. Research also shows that garlic may help in preventing various types of cancer and diabetes.

Garlic also has blood thinning properties. If someone is already on anticoagulant drugs, consuming excessive amounts of garlic might not be advised. Because of this, I strongly advise seeking medical advice before taking garlic supplements. Though, honestly, it's so versatile and tasty, I'm not sure a pill form is really required.

During my treatment phase, no savoury dish I consumed was without garlic. On the rare occasion where I could eat salads, I would combine garlic powder with olive oil and lemon juice for a quick dressing.

While I didn't notice any immediately obvious physical benefits after eating garlic, it certainly made my meals more palatable. Ginger may have immediately quelled my nausea, but garlic just made my life better. Truth.

How to use it:

The best way to release the healthy compounds in garlic is to crush or mince the cloves a few minutes before adding them to any dish. Any form of garlic is potent and works as powerfully as raw garlic. So powdered or dried garlic is great too. Pre-minced garlic, the kind you find in a jar at the supermarket, has been stored for a long time, losing all its flavour and its nutritional value. The soaking liquid is mostly water, though sometimes they'll add phosphoric acid, which is not good for you.

When I didn't feel like a lengthy meal, I would boil some pasta, chop some garlic, and add the chopped garlic to a pan with good quality olive oil, salt, and pepper. It's a delicious meal on its own. I always overdo it on the garlic, because I love it so much. How much you use is really up to you; a couple cloves should do.

For an easy snack, remove the outer layer of skin on a bulb of garlic, keep the cloves intact. Cut off the top bit to expose some of the garlic inside and drizzle the entire bulb with olive oil. Wrap it in aluminium foil and roast it in the over for about 20 minutes. Once baked, the garlic will squeeze out very easily. The now soft garlic and be mushed into a paste that you can spread on toast, or combine it with tahini and yogurt to make a healthy dip.

GINGER | *ADHUWA* | *ADHRAK*

A staple in any Asian household, ginger is not only used in Ayurvedic medicine but is common among traditional Chinese medicines as well. It has many powerful nutrients and an unmistakable flavour profile.

Benefits:

During chemotherapy, ginger (and Himalayan rock salt) rescued me from my terrible nausea spells. It's a miracle root for nausea and has also been hailed as a way to combat migraines. Gingerol, the compound that gives ginger all its goodness, smell, and taste, is an anti-inflammatory and a powerful antioxidant. It also helped me with the major indigestion I faced during my treatment.

How to use it:

There are so many ways to use ginger in whichever way you fancy. Honestly, your "fancies" during chemotherapy are few and far between, so just pick whatever's simplest.

These are the ways I used to (and still do) incorporate ginger:

1. Grate a thumb-sized piece of ginger into 250 ml of water. Leave it to infuse for half an hour, strain, and drink. You can use warm water or cold. Adding honey is always an option, if you fancy something sweet.

2. Cut or shred ginger into small bits, sprinkle Himalayan rock salt on it. You could also use *kala namark* or *bire-noon*; the smell might be pungent but it really helps. Let the ginger dry out. Either pop it into the oven on a low heat or dry it out in the sun. If you own a dehydrator, that'll be your best bet. Store it in an airtight container, popping a few pieces in a baggie in your purse. Pop some in your mouth when the nausea hits.

3. Simply chew on smaller pieces of raw ginger for extreme nausea. Try not to leave it pressed up against your cheeks or gums for too long - the natural juices are very strong and can cause some damage.

4. Make homemade ginger ale by boiling 1 ½ cups of peeled and chopped ginger with 2 cups water,

along with 1 cup of sugar/agave/ honey or any natural sugar substitute. Let it simmer on low heat for half an hour. The result will be a thick, sweet ginger syrup. Much like a cordial. Strain the syrup and store it in the fridge for a few days. When the mood strikes, pour around 50ml of the ginger syrup into a glass and top it up with sparkling water. It's the tastiest way to sip away your nausea.

I don't think there is such a thing as too much ginger but, like anything else, eat what your body and mind might feel like, don't over-do anything. If you want to take a ginger supplement, then speak to someone who would know more about the quantity recommended.

HIMALAYAN BLACK ROCK SALT | *BIRE-NOON | KALA-NAMAK*

Yet another staple in a Nepali Kitchen is black salt.

Rock salt contains minerals which normal sea salt does not. Most table salt widely used today contains more sodium than rock salt. Rock salt is high in calcium, magnesium, iron and many other minerals, overall making it the healthier version of salts. As the name suggests it comes from rocks and in the Himalayas. The most common rock salt available in the market is the one which is pink in colour, but there is another version that is used in South Asian cuisine, black rock salt.

Black salt is another type of rock salt commonly found in the Himalayas and widely used within this region.Because it is high in sulfur, it has a strange strange smell and taste. While regular Himalyan rock salt is mostly pinkish in colour, black salt is dark red or black in colour. Every time I open the jar of black salt at home, it smells.. well... a little farty. Apologies for the unappealing description, but it does. Despite the smell, it does taste just like regular salt.

Benefits:

Black salt is known to aid digestion. If you ever visit India, a common drink you will find is lemon soda, which is basically lime juice with soda water. You get it in three variations: sweet (with sugar syrup), salt (with black salt), and mix of sugar and salt. Commonly used as an electrolyte solution, people are encouraged to drink it during summer. The drink is also alkaline, so it's great for settling the stomach before or after a spice-heavy Indian meal.

The laxative properties in black salt make it a great weight loss aid. Rich in potassium, black salt is also good for muscle cramps and spasms. It's an all 'round helpful seasoning to keep in the pantry, for sure.

How to use it:

Black salt isn't commonly used in food preparation because of its powerful smell. It is, however, widely used in drinks, some sauté salads, and chaats. While it works great with lemon soda water, it can also be added to dry roasted cumin powder and water to make another very refreshing drink.

TAMARIND | *IMLI*

When I was younger, we often travelled to Thailand very often on holiday. With more than a few friends living there, we spent a lot of time near the Myanmar/ Thai border. It was a prime spot for children (myself included) to steal fresh young coconuts and tamarind pods from our neighbours' trees.

To reach the coconuts, we tied a small sharp knife to the end of a long stick, and from our balcony, we slowly severed the branch that was attached to the fruit. Two friends would be standing below with a bed sheet we stole from one of the rooms to catch the coconut as it fell, and to make sure it didn't crack open on the floor, spilling that sweet coconut water inside. For tamarind, we split the end of the stick by a few centimeters and used it to grab hold of the branch holding the fresh tamarind. Then we would rotate and rotate and rotate before the branch broke off from the main tree.

We'd spend the next while enjoying our booty; getting our hands and faces filthy and sticky with absolutely no regrets.

Thinking back, I'm not sure how I managed to enjoy something so sour. I mean, occasionally, you'd luck out with a sweet-ish pod, but for the most part they really made your lips pucker. Maybe it had more to do with the adrenaline rush and the cheeky fun of it all than the actual flavour.

If you're unfamiliar with tamarind, it's the edible fruit of a massive (leguminous) tree indigenous to Africa. It's widely consumed in many parts of Asian and Latin America too. Have you ever had *chaat*, or *pani puri* in an Indian restaurant? That muddy brown liquid or thick brown tangy sauce is what tamarind is. It is also used in Caribbean, Mexican, and other Latin American cultures to make candies.

If all of the above seems unfamiliar and you think you have never tried tamarind, think again. It's one of the main ingredients in original Worcestershire Sauce and HP sauce.

Tamarind is high in tartaric acid, which makes it extremely sour. The pulp also contains high levels of calcium, B vitamins, niacin, and thiamine. This makes tamarind not just a flavour booster, but also amazing at fighting infections, fever, and digestive problems.

Although a rare find, I have spotted tamarind paste at many supermarkets around London. It's definitely something you'll find in an Indian grocery store. Always read the instructions on the label, because it comes in various forms. The dry and pressed pulp, found in most Indian stores, is probably the easiest to use. Dilute a small piece of the pulp with warm water, then drain and press through a sieve. Keep an eye out for seeds that need to be discarded - they're not small enough for you to want to end up with one in your mouth.

Use it when cooking curries, or even in Daal. It gives a zingy kick that pumps up the flavour of your food from 20 to 100. The delicious tangy flavour makes food more appealing. With all the benefits of tamarind, you're hitting two birds with one stone.

I made a drink with tamarind when I had to hydrate and flush the medication out of my system more aggressively than usual. Homemade variations of lemonade, ginger ale or other drinks are far better for someone than the drinks you might find on a grocery store shelf.

My cousin shared a great hack with me - a quick frozen snack to cool the mouth and get those appetite-boosting enzymes flowing. Just freeze some tamarind with a pinch of salt and sugar, and grab a lolly when the mood strikes.

TURMERIC | BESAR | HALDI

Turmeric is my favorite spice. With an endless list of nutritional benefits and amazing anti-inflammatory properties, it's an all-round winner. Although commonly used in household and kitchen applications since I can remember, my obsession is just recent.

In 2013, while living in New-Delhi, I began to suffer from uncomfortable rashes and pimples on my face and arms. After multiple dermatologist appointments and buying expensive French face-washes and tubes of medical-grade creams, there were no signs of improvement. It was certainly not pollution. I had changed my diet, so it was certainly not what I was eating.

My husband recommended I speak with his family physician. Very hesitant, yet with nothing to lose, I decided to speak with him and share images of my condition. I later received a text from Dr. S, with the names of two over-the-counter, all-natural medicines that I needed to take for 15 days. After about 2 weeks I began to see my skin clear and I was intrigued by what these tablets were. One was Curcuma Longa L. (turmeric) and the other Piper Nigrum L. (black pepper). My obsession took hold then and there.

A root of a flowering plant that belongs to the ginger family, turmeric is often used in its dried and powdered form. Incredibly versatile in foods and as natural remedies, it's become one of my absolute favourite pantry staples.

Although most beneficial when used raw, when I tried to consume small pieces of turmeric root, I stained my teeth, my hands, and my knife. The taste of raw turmeric is also incredibly strong, maybe even too strong, even for someone who's been using it throughout their lives. The powder is almost as powerful as the fresh root - which makes it a great addition to any kitchen cupboard. It has super anti-inflammatory properties and is an absolute boss at fighting infection.

Benefits:

Turmeric helps with body pain, teeth and gum problems, insect bites, and more. I most recently used turmeric on my pierced ear lobe. Because of its powerful anti-bacterial properties, turmeric is known to reduce disease-causing bacterial growth inside our bodies. It also combats bacterial growth on the surface, when used as a facepack or applied over cuts or bruises.

How to use it:

I am not a medical professional, so if you're looking for more professional advice I would suggest contacting a physician if your concerns are deeply medical. I try to use turmeric in my food as often as I can. Sometimes I'll add half a teaspoon (or less) to smoothies, or soups. It gives a lovely colour but the taste can be overpowering if you add too much.

For injuries or other external purposes, you can always get information on websites. I usually mix it with raw mustard oil or pure olive oil to make a thick paste to apply to the affected area.

NOTE: When using turmeric in food, always - yes, always - add freshly ground black pepper. The properties of curcumin works ten times better and becomes more potent if combined with pepper. This can be a tiny amount, just a pinch.

Too much of anything is never a good thing. If you consume too much turmeric, whether as a supplement or as an ingredient, then your iron absorption is much slower than it should be.

JIMBU AND TIMUR

These two spices are very rare and typical to Nepali cuisine. No black *daal* is made without *Jimbu* and no tomato *ko achaar* will go without a sprinkling of *timur*.

Jimbu

Jimbu belongs to the onion family. It tastes a bit like a cross between spring onion and chives. It is almost always used in its dried herb form. It is one of the herbs that might not have a very versatile use in everyday cooking, but when it comes to tempering *daals*, especially black *daal*, it is absolutely essential. Some people also use *Jimbu* in curries, soups, and meat dishes. The dried herb is added to hot oil or ghee to revive its natural flavour and fragrance.

The use of *Jimbu* originates from the northern mountainous region of Nepal. Its use is more frequent due to the cold climate. Medicinally, it helps with flu symptoms. It is boiled in water and then drunk to help with coughs, colds, and flu.

It's not easy to find *Jimbu* in any Asian stores in London or other major global cities. Having said that, there are some online portals that sell Nepali spices and herbs where you can probably spot *Jimbu*.

Timur

Often referred to as the "spice of Nepal", *Timur* is cultivated in the Himalayan region of Nepal during September/October. It grows in clusters like tiny berries, which are then dried. As a dried berry, it has a mild and citrusy scent. The aroma intensifies a hundred fold once it is ground into powder form. It can be used in both forms.

Timur comes from the same family as Szechuan peppercorns, which are used widely in Chinese (Szechuan/ Sichuan) cuisine. On its own, Timur is spicy enough to numb the tongue.

It can be used in almost any dish; meat, vegetables, salads (achaar), soups and most tomato based dishes benefit from a pinch or two of *Timur.* The heat in this spice helps tenderise meat, while keeping it juicy. A tiny bit goes a long long way too.

A common way of using *timur* is to make what we call *chhop.* *Timur ko chhop* is made by using coriander seeds, cumin seeds, *timur* seeds, roasted and blended with dry chillies and salt. It can be consumed on its own or added to other dishes and condiments.

Timur is considered to be good for freshening up your breath and for battling common toothache. It is also a good remedy for colds, coughs, head and stomach aches. It is a natural anti-inflammatory since it contains phytosterols and terpenes, both of which are antioxidants. *Timur* also contains a significant amount of potassium which is good for cardio-vascular health.

If you can't find Nepali *Timur* in supermarkets, Sichuan peppercorns make a great substitute.

Every culture, every tradition has its own set of home remedies that have been passed down from one generation to the next. Over time, we have forgotten to use them. They have been given less importance since the advancement of pharmaceutical drugs.

Pharmaceutical drugs are cutting-edge and life-saving. Medical advancements in the last few decades have been phenomenal. If I had cancer some 50 years ago, I would have not lived to see this day. I am forever grateful to modern science and technology.

However, I firmly believe that we can integrate the old traditional home remedies on a daily basis. We can avoid taking paracetamol when we have a toothache,when there is clove oil nearby.

With the help of the internet and our grandparents, grand uncles and aunts, we have access to a pool of knowledge that was used long before pharmaceutical drugs became the order of the day.

Herbs and spices might not be able to completely cure chronic conditions, but they can certainly help in many other ways. Ayurvedic treatments, one of the oldest medicines in the world, is completely based on what comes from the earth.

My trust in natural remedies helped me cope with chemotherapy a little better. The variety of food in my own culture, and other cultures, gave me options to choose from. When I didn't have an appetite for some I opted for another.

I was always focusing on eating, gaining my strength, and fighting the disease.

RECIPES

FRESH AND HEALTHY - LIKE MY GRANDMOTHER WOULD MAKE

12 August 2016, my first day of chemotherapy.

As we were about to leave for the hospital, a package was delivered - a surprise from my husband. It was a book, personally signed and with a note from my favourite chef, Jamie Oliver, which his team had been kind enough to send.

When I saw it, I cried. It was one of the few moments in my life where I cried true tears of joy. It is also one of the most thoughtful and adorable gifts I have ever received. My husband has always appreciated and encouraged my fondness for food and cooking.

While I was going through the treatment process, I tried to find books that would help me prepare simple meals, without much hassle. The lack of energy and appetite alone were enough to dissuade anyone from eating or cooking. I was extremely fortunate that my mother had come to my rescue, from over 7000km away.

Eating stale food is not recommended, so fresh meals had to be prepared every time. (Or frozen shortly after preparation.) During my treatment, my mother cooked at least three times a day, if not more. I think she cooked more in those six months than she had my entire life - I guess the love for their children can motivate mothers to move mountains. She wouldn't even let me pick up my own plate, let alone cook or wash the dishes.

Though I found numerous recipe books detailing what I could eat as a cancer patient, written by medical professionals, nutritionists, and superb chefs around the globe, I couldn't find one that my palate could relate to. As a South Asian, I grew up with dishes that featured over 50 spices, and I like my rice. Soup for every meal just doesn't cut it for me.

I followed a few tips from some amazing bloggers who had gone through the same journey as me, but most of what I ate came at the recommendation of my family - my grandmothers, grand aunts, aunts and uncles, and the families of those aunts and uncles. You get it if you're a desi.

In the beginning, you might be sick and might not be able to stomach anything, but eventually, your appetite returns. You get hungry and can have cravings. My fridge was always full of food - I never knew when I wanted to eat, or what.

At the same time, there were days when my father or my husband would have to finish my meals, since I wasn't in the mood for anything. My mother called it the 'garbage moment'.

Here, I would like to share some recipes of the healthy and flavourful foods that helped me to tackle the nausea, and gave me strength to wake up each morning.

A FEW "FAMILY SECRETS"

I'm adding two of the most precious (and best kept) family secrets in a section of their own. Both of these are cupboard staples - they belong in every home. These are incredibly special to me and I'm proud to share them here.

Ma's Healing Powder

My grandmother, Ma, is who I'll call if I need help when I feel unwell. She's a wealth of all sorts of herbal remedies. She taught me the benefits of turmeric and mustard oil, and she is also the one who also always reminded us that there are times you can do with-out pharmaceutical medicines.

In the summer of 1992, I clearly remember going on one of our family road trips. Like any other desi family trips, ours included, mum, dad, grandmother, grandfather, my dad's sister, my mother's sister and her two daughters, my grandfather's cousin, and one neighbour whom we also called "Uncle". (We call any one who is our parent's age (or older) "uncle" or "aunty".)

One of my cousins always had frequent nausea (motion sickness or otherwise) which got worse on road trips. Ma gave her a small box of smelly powder, a pinch of which always seemed to help. My cousin would swirl this dusty remedy around in her mouth and her headaches and sweats would go away. We had no idea what was in that powder but it was clear that whichever spices she used had some kind of healing power.

I now know that the farty smell was because of the high sulphur content in black salt. It wasn't so great to have it wafting around a van, cramped up with so many people. But I don't mind the smell too much now.

Years later, I asked Ma for the recipe of this miracle powder. It dawned on me that we didn't know what was in it. Everytime we needed some, Ma always prepared it and sent it over. Of course, she wouldn't share the finer details with me, but she did give me an idea of what was in it. When, however, I announced that I wanted to include it in this book, she was happy to share it.

This powder is not something you will get used to easily. It smells and tastes extremely strong. All the ingredients in it have amazing healing properties and honestly, it was probably one of the more powerful things that helped with my nausea when I was going through chemo. It also helped my stomach relax after throwing up every hour for 8 hours, after those more intense treatment sessions.

Ingredients:

- 2 tablespoons black salt (If you can't find black salt, you can use Himalayan rock salt)
- ½ tablespoon *jwano* or *ajwain* powder
- ½ tablespoon fennel seeds powder
- 1 tablespoon dry mint leaf powder
- Pinch of *timur* (optional)

Combine all the ingredients and store in a jar. Only use a small pinch at a time. It's quite potent and salty, so you really won't need a lot.

Mamu's Garam Masala

This is my mom's special garam masala. I have been using it my whole life without realising that it wasn't store bought. I used to think it was the 'Nepali' garam masala. When I asked my mom if she could find out what's in it, she laughed.

I use this whether I am making something sweet, savory, or even drinks. It's a simple concoction of 4 spices, with fifth one being totally optional.

It contains:

1. Green cardamom
2. Clove
3. Cinnamon
4. Black cardamom
5. Long pepper fruit, or *Pipra* in Nepali (optional if you can't find any)

To make this garam masala powder, you need each of these in powder form. Mix a tablespoon of all the four ingredients and store it in a jar. If you wish to add the *Pipra*, it should be exactly half of all the other spices. So if you have used one tablespoon of clove, cardamom, cinnamon, and black cardamom, then use only half a tablespoon of the *Pipra*. This mixture will last at least six months, or less if you are like me and use it often.

Here's how I use it:

Add ½ teaspoon of this spice mix to a cup of hot boiling water, add honey and enjoy it as a soothing drink, especially if you have a cold or bad cough. You can always add ginger and or lemon to this combination too.

Add ½ teaspoon to some warm milk (or milk alternative of your choice) along with turmeric, black pepper, a few strands of saffron, and honey. Simmer until everything's mixed up well. This is the best golden milk you'll ever try. It not only helps you get a good night's sleep, but if you have it regularly when you know you might feel ill, it will keep your immune system up and infection at bay.

Sprinkle it on plain yogurt and add honey if you are ever craving something sweet. It's like a dessert on its own - trust me. A pinch or two in some rice pudding works wonders too!

If you are making any vegetable curry, add it towards the end of the cooking process to amp up the flavors a bit. It works just as well in soups and stews. A good heaping spoonful will help to tenderise meat, so add it when you want to keep your meal juicy and flavourful.

RECIPES

I am no chef. I have absolutely no knife skills, although I really wish I did. One thing I've always wanted is to be able to chop like a chef. I cook the way our grandmothers did, making use of the five senses: smell, sight, taste, touch and, believe it or not, hearing.

I don't think it's just me, either. On the cooking shows I watch, I often notice the chefs listening to their food - they can hear the sizzle when their food burns, or the lack of crackle that says the pan is not hot enough. In many South Asian households, the use of a pressure cooker is common. My mother would often give me instructions for a recipe, and she would mention how many whistles to listen for before the meal is ready.

That's what it means to listen to your food being prepared. Even with boiling water, it's not just the sight of the water that tells you if you've used too much heat, or too little. It's also the sound.

In cooking, the degree of heat you use is important - the integrity of the food depends on it. Food cooked on a low heat is often better than on a high heat. While it is, of course, convenient because it cooks faster, your food may need more time than the high heat gives. This is also why pots that are thick, or have a thick base, are better to cook in, because they retain heat. For all my recipes, I recommend cooking in a deep dish pan.

For me, it's important to get my hands dirty while I cook. Using your hands can give you a good idea of the texture of the food, before it reaches your mouth. If you ever make *aaloo ko achaar* or cold glass noodles, you can get an idea of the consistency just by mixing it with your hands. The perfect combination of oil and lemon or vinegar can be felt between your fingertips.

They say that you get weird cravings during pregnancy - those are nothing compared to the side effects of chemotherapy or radiotherapy. Some days, your appetite is out of control. Others, everything tastes awful.

During chemo, I craved a lot of spicy food - food that tasted sour, with little or no sweetness. I was never a vegetarian and I grew up in a meat-eating culture. With the chemo, I couldn't even smell, let alone eat, meat or eggs. My favourite dishes, such as *momo*, made mostly with meat, or *biryani*, the only dish my husband makes perfectly, seemed like a distant dream.

Worse was the smell of anything sweet.

Have you ever binged on sugar, like chocolates, ice-creams, or cakes, only to have your stomach tell you it was a bad idea before your mind does?

The safest option for me was savoury food, with some spice.

One thing to keep in mind before we get to the recipes: A person undergoing treatment may not want to eat any of the recipes I cover. They may also find the sound of the recipe appealing at first, only to change their mind when the dish is put in front of them.

> *Dear caretakers, please don't take offense at*
> *the rejection of your hard work and cooking.*
> *They can't help it.*

Another thing to remember is that every cancer case is different. So are the side-effects, taste buds, and appetite during this time. By preparing multiple dishes, and keeping them in the fridge or freezer, you can give them the option to eat what they want, if they want to. In this case, it's better to have more than less. Though do remember, fresher is better, so don't store the food for too long!

This is where friends and family members who offer to help come in handy. When your friends and family ask what they can do to help, stop being a brave soul, and ask them to prepare some of the dishes below. Trust me, people who offer to help actually want to help and be a part of your life. Give them that opportunity.

Below, I have listed some of the dishes I ate during my treatment. Some, I continue to eat and some I know are very good when you are feeling unwell - whether from side-effects, a cold or the flu, or a bad stomach. Even if you just feel like eating something hearty, you can refer to these and whip something up.

These are not my recipes. They are age-old. I've just jotted them down as they are some of the foods I (and many others) eat for their healing and comforting properties because they are packed with good nutrients.

PULSES & LEGUMES

1. JAULO (KHICHADI)

Jaulo is basically a variation of Indian *Khichadi*. Though it uses different ingredients and has a different consistency, the result is almost the same. Most babies eat a lot of *Jaulo*, because it is healthy, with natural carbohydrates and proteins, and it's easy for their stomachs to digest. It's like a lazy person's comfort food - just put everything in a pan and cook it until it comes together.

Rich in protein and carbohydrates, with plenty of vitamins, fibre, and so on, *Jaulo* is ideal for those going through cancer treatment, as it is easy to swallow and won't take too much time and effort to chew. Using very few spices, it's also soothing to the stomach, especially for those who have sensitive stomachs or who may develop gastritis during this time. I did, of course.

Ingredients:

- ½ cup (100g) rice
- 1 cup *daal* (200g) - ideally (split) *Moong daal*, though you can use others (or combine some varieties)
- 1 teaspoon oil or *ghee*
- 2 -3 cups (600ml) water
- 1 teaspoon turmeric
- 2 - 3 cloves garlic
- A pinch of *hing* (*asafoetida*)
- Salt and pepper to taste
- *Optional:* Vegetables, such as onions, green beans, tomatoes, as well as any other spices - as many or as few as you'd like. This recipe is usually kept

basic and simple because it's best to avoid overly spicy or oily food during this time

Directions:

Soak the rice and *daal* before you start cooking. They don't require a lot of soaking time, and can be soaked together.

Add oil or *ghee* to a warm pan or pressure cooker. Once the oil warms up, add garlic. Saute the garlic on medium heat until golden brown and fragrant. Add *hing*, turmeric, and black pepper. As the spices begin to sizzle, drain the rice and *daal*, saving the water they have been soaked in.

Mix in the *daal* and rice, stirring every 2 to 3 minutes, letting the mixture dry before adding the soaking water. Add up to 2 ½ cups.

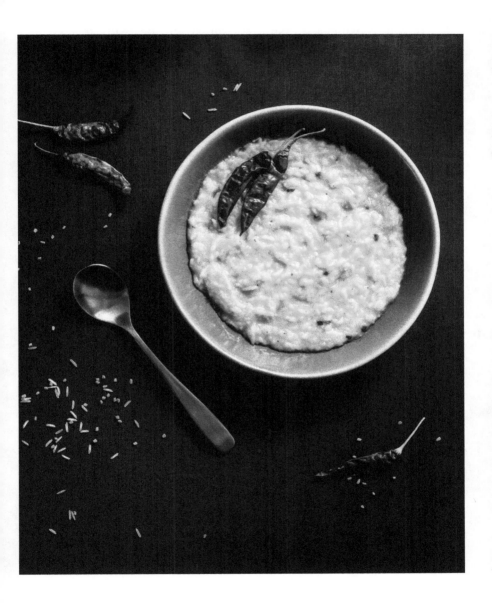

Cover and cook for another 20 minutes on low heat.

If you're using a pressure cooker, it will be ready in less time - just 2 or 3 whistles.

The consistency should be mushy, though you should be able to see the rice and *daal*. It should be soft enough that everything comes together to make a thick stew.

Add a bit of lemon before serving, sprinkle with some freshly chopped coriander leaves, and enjoy - or rather, eat just to heal.

Note:

Most true desi will have a pressure cooker in their kitchen. If you don't, and if you're not a desi, you can always use a saucepan. Make sure it's big enough to hold double the volume of all the ingredients, because as rice and *daal* cook, they double in size.

2. QWATI

Qwati is a stew made with nine sprouted beans. While it can be prepared anytime, in Nepal, almost every household prepares it on *Janai Purnima* - the same day as *Rakhi*, for Indians - which usually falls in August, and always on the full moon. It marks the end of summer and the start of monsoon.

The beans used in the stew are: black gram, green gram, chickpea, field bean, soybean, field pea, garden pea, cowpea, and rice bean.

Because of the variety of beans, and the fact that they are sprouted, this dish is packed with nutrients. It is known to cure a cold, keep you warm during the changing weather, and is good for women who are pregnant and breastfeeding.

I have been told that the best way to sprout the beans is to soak them in cold water for at least 2 hours, before draining them and leaving them lightly covered with a muslin cloth, somewhere dark and away from direct sunlight. I've always found it an impossible task to sprout things. I either add too much water, or too little, or I leave it alone for days on end. It explains why I am terrible at gardening.

Mixed sprouted beans, which are now readily available in many supermarkets, are a good alternative to soaking and sprouting them at home. Unfortunately, these mixes do not include the sprouted alfalfa or mung beans. To make a good *Qwati*, you must have a variety of sprouted beans.

Ingredients:

- 300g soaked and sprouted mixed beans
- 1 large potato
- 2 or 3 medium tomatoes
- 120g onions
- 12g ginger
- 18g garlic
- 2g *jwano*
- ½ teaspoon coriander powder
- ½ teaspoon cumin powder
- ⅓ teaspoon turmeric
- Salt and pepper to taste
- Optional: 2g *rai* (mustard seed)

Directions:

Heat a pan, add oil and temper it with some *jwano*. Add the potatoes and let them brown before adding the ginger, garlic, and onion. Mix well and sauté for another 5 to 10 minutes.

Add the soaked, sprouted mixed beans, along with turmeric powder, coriander and cumin powder. Let this simmer for a bit before creating space in the centre of the pan and adding the tomatoes. Cover the tomatoes with the other ingredients and let the mixture cook for 5 minutes. The tomatoes will begin to release water. Mix everything well, before adding salt and pepper to taste, along with about 4 cups of water.

Lower the heat and cook, covered, for 30 to 40 minutes. If you are using a pressure cooker, 10 minutes in the pressure cooker should do. The dish is ready when the biggest grain sprout or potato can be smoothly and easily smashed against your spoon.

You can adjust the consistency by adding more water to thin it out, or thicken by cooking it without the lid.

Qwati is best enjoyed with rice, but it can be a meal on its own.

Tip: Add a dollop of Greek yoghurt and a sprinkle of mint for the perfect meal.

3. *Daal (Dal)*

To me, *daal* is like a warm bowl of hugs and cuddles. If prepared correctly, all you need is some rice, bread, or *naan* for dipping, and you have a good meal.

In Nepal, we prepare *daal* differently than in other parts of South Asia. Each *daal* in the region is unique, and tastes as good as the other. In Bangladesh, I ate a delicious *daal* with eggs and fish. In India, *daal* is as rich as its other dishes, cooked with tomatoes and onions. In Pakistan, *daal* is aromatic and has the creamiest texture, served with fried onions on top.

In Nepal, *daal* is more like a clear soup than a stew. We also only use ginger and turmeric for almost all *daals*, tempering it with *ghee* and cumin, and sometimes adding garlic at the end. The dish varies from one family to another. Everyone has their own version and preparation method, making it unique. Even if you've had enough of your own *daal*, you can easily enjoy a bowl at someone else's home, because it will taste completely different.

Daal is made with dried, split or whole pulses or legumes. There are many varieties of *daal*. While the French use Puy lentils in salads or fish, and Turkish soups are usually lentil-based, I think that the Indian subcontinent has mastered cooking lentils.

We have a *daal* for every illness. There is *daal* for when you have fever, *daal* for when you are injured, to help you gain strength and heal faster. There is a *daal* for kidney stones and a *daal* for when your stomach aches. No dinner or lunch is complete without some *daal*.

I am sharing the recipes for two types of *daal*, though the same rules can be applied to all other *daals*. You can also jazz them up by adding some vegetables or greens of your choice to make a nice stew.

MUNG OR MUSURO (MASOOR)

For this recipe, you can use either *mung* or *musuro daal.* *Moong,* or *mung* split *daal* is yellow in colour, while *musuro* is almost reddish. They are both very good for when someone is unwell. They give a boost of energy and help you heal a lot faster, making you stronger.

Ingredients:

Serves 4

- 1 cup lentils
- 4 to 4 ½ cups of water
- 1 teaspoon *ghee*
- ½ teaspoon cumin seeds
- ¾ teaspoon ginger
- ¼ teaspoon turmeric powder
- Salt to taste

If you do not have a pressure cooker, it's best to cook this in a thick pot, because it needs to simmer for a long time. If not using a pressure cooker, you should rinse the lentils and soak them for about an hour before cooking

Directions

Add the turmeric, ginger, salt, water and lentils to a pan. Simmer and cook for about 40 minutes to an hour, or until the lentils are soft to the touch. You can also mash some to make them smooth.

Tempering is optional, but is recommended, as it adds and seals in flavour.

To Temper:

You can use *ghee* or coconut oil. Once the *ghee* is hot, add cumin seeds. Once the cumin begins to change colour, pour this over the *daal*. It will make a sizzling sound, but this is normal. You can also add chopped spring onions at the end, to the oil/*ghee* as an added "flavour bomb" which goes so well with this *daal*.

Serve hot with rice. Your body will thank you

BLACK DAAL

There is something about *Kaalo* (black) *daal* that feels like home. *Kaalo daal* with *saag* and *golbeda ko achaar* is the ultimate warm hug. The taste is so simple, yet it brings back so many memories.

In India, black *daal* is totally different. It is either full or without the husk, often cooked with cream, butter, and spices. In Nepal, all we need is ginger to create a taste that's out of this world.

Black *daal* is prepared the same way as the other *daals*. The difference is that it is usually cooked in a cast-iron dish, making it very rich in iron. Modern households use a pressure cooker, which is certainly not made of cast iron, so they drop a ring of cast iron into the pot while cooking, giving the daal an added boost of flavour.

Black lentil skin can surface while the *daal* is being cooked, making a slight foam. It's quite easy to skim it off, since it all floats to the top. Don't be alarmed if you find black *daal* slimier than other *daals*. That's where it gets its creamier texture from.

Ingredients:

- 1 cup black *daal*
- 4 to 4 ½ cups of water
- 1 teaspoon ginger
- Salt to taste

To Temper

- 1 teaspoon *ghee*
- ½ teaspoon *jimbu*

Combine all the ingredients and cook the same way as described above. If you don't want to temper, just add a big teaspoon of *ghee* towards the end. *Ghee* and black *daal* go together very well, and are like a match made in heaven when eaten with a warm bowl of steamed rice.

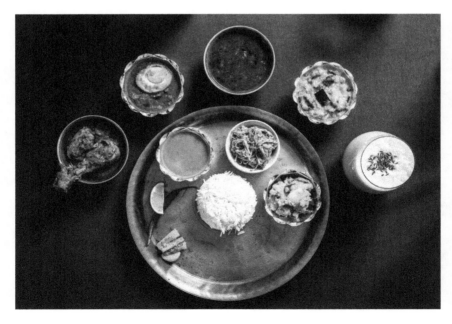

4. JWANO KO JHOL

In Nepal, our meals will usually include one carbohydrate - mostly rice or *roti* - a *daal* and some vegetables, along with meat and a condiment. As an alternative to *daal*, we also have a variety of *jhols*. Almost like a cross between a soup and a stew, *jhol* can be very clear and soup-like, or thick and stew-like.

This dish may shock you at first, because of the quantity of *jwano* we use, but the overpowering taste of garlic, cumin, and coriander powder transforms this *jhol* into a bowl of healing goodness.

Jwano - *ajwain* in Hindi - is particularly good for the digestive system. When I was younger and had a bad stomach ache, my grandmother would chew on some *jwano* - probably to release the oils in the seeds - and then put it around my belly button.

When I had digestive issues, *jhol* was the best meal I could have had. It soothed my stomach and calmed my entire digestive tract.

Ingredients:

- 4 large cloves of garlic, crushed
- 2 tablespoons *jwano* (*ajwain*)
- 1 teaspoon *ghee*
- ½ teaspoon ginger
- ½ teaspoon cumin (*jeera*) powder
- ½ teaspoon coriander (*dhaniya*) powder
- ¼ teaspoon turmeric
- Salt to taste

Directions:

Heat some *ghee* in a pan. Once warm, add garlic and let it brown a little. Once the garlic is slightly browned, add the *jwano* to the pan. Mix and let the *jwano* change colour and become fragrant.

Add the turmeric, cumin, and coriander powder. Mix evenly and add two cups of water. Bring to a boil and add salt and ginger. Boil down to your preferred consistency and serve with rice.

5. *BESAN KO KADI* - *CHICKPEA FLOUR STEW*

In my opinion, this recipe was stolen from Indian Punjabi food, and Nepali-fied. It was not until I started living in India, and married a Punjabi, that I ate the best *royal kadhi.*

The use of chickpeas is very common in Nepal, so this recipe is not the Punjabi version. It is simple and easy to make and doesn't have *pakoda*. I loved the fact that, even when I was weak and unable to do intensive cooking, making a *kadi* was quick, easy, and delicious. At this point, I had had enough of *daal* and needed a different source of protein.

This recipe calls for yoghurt, but it can also be made with water instead, for a vegan option.

Ingredients:

- 1 cup *besan* (chickpea flour)
- 2 cups plain, non-Greek yoghurt, mixed with water to a thin, almost buttermilk-like consistency
- 1 to 3 green chillies, depending on your spice preference

- 5 to 7 curry leaves
- ½ teaspoon turmeric
- ½ teaspoon *jeera* (cumin seed)
- ½ teaspoon mustard seed
- Salt to taste
- Oil

Directions:

In a mixing bowl, combine *besan* and thinned yoghurt with a whisk. Add water until it reaches a thin, water-like consistency.

Heat the oil in a pan, and add mustard seeds. Once the seeds begin to pop and dance all over your pan, add the cumin seeds. When those change colour, add the curry leaves, turmeric, and green chillies. After they become fragrant, add the liquids.

As the *besan* boils, it will become thick and you may have to add more water. Let the mixture boil for 15 to 20 minutes, mixing continuously, as it can thicken and stick. I like to use a whisk. Keep adding water until it reaches your preferred consistency. Taste and add salt if more is required.

Kadi should be slightly on the sour side. While the yoghurt should add a natural sourness, you can also add a dash of lemon or lime juice at the end. This dish is best enjoyed with rice.

CURRY DISHES

Curry powder plays an important role for those who are fond of cooking Indian food. Despite this, I don't usually recommend curry powder. If you go to India and ask for curry powder, they'll probably laugh at you - and they won't understand what you're looking for. Each curry has its own spice.

Different spices should be added at different times, and in different quantities. Using a spoonful of mixed spices all at the same might leave some spices uncooked, some overcooked and others tasting strange.

Seeds should go in first, followed by turmeric, which requires a bit more cooking time. Cumin and coriander powder often go together, like best friends, and some spices should be added towards the end.

6. *PALUNGA KO JHOL* - *SPINACH CURRY*

Ingredients:

- 4 cups of spinach, finely chopped
- 3 to 4 cloves garlic, crushed
- 1 large tomato, chopped
- 1 tablespoon vegetable oil
- ½ teaspoon ginger
- ¼ teaspoon turmeric
- Salt to taste

Directions:

Add garlic to a pan of warm oil. Once the garlic begins to change colour, add tomatoes and cook for a few more minutes until the tomatoes start to soften. Add turmeric and mix evenly, then add spinach. Mix the spinach around to coat the flavours of tomatoes and garlic. Then add water and let it boil until it reaches your desired consistency.

7. AALOO KO JHOL - POTATO CURRY

This is my home in a bowl. A comforting food, the taste takes me back to a time when there would be religious events at home, and we needed to make food without garlic and onion.

Garlic and onions are aphrodisiac foods, so during religious events, making 'pure' food means cooking without these two main ingredients of Nepali/Indian cooking. This recipe calls for both onion and garlic.

The aromatic smell of potatoes and tomatoes, often enjoyed with *roti* or *puri* (fried bread), or over a warm bowl of rice is nothing but satisfying. The tiny bits of *jeera* (cumin) makes the experience even more adventurous. The garnish of coriander is perfect harmony. And who on this planet doesn't like potatoes?

Note:

For any curry, you can adjust the consistency by adding more or less water, depending on your preference.

Ingredients:

Serves two

- 4 medium potatoes, chopped into big chunks
- 1 onion, finely chopped
- 2 - 3 cloves of garlic
- 2 medium tomatoes, chopped
- 1 teaspoon coriander powder
- 1 tablespoon oil
- ½ teaspoon cumin seeds
- ½ teaspoon cumin powder
- ½ teaspoon turmeric
- Salt to taste
- Coriander to garnish

Directions:

Heat a deep dish or heavy-based, deep saucepan. Add the oil and then the cumin seeds once the oil is hot. You will notice a crackling sound and a change in colour. Once the seeds darken, but before they burn, add the onions. Saute on medium heat until the onions soften, and then add the garlic. Let the garlic sweat before adding the potatoes.

Allow the potatoes to brown a bit, add the turmeric, and mix. Give it a few more minutes, and then push everything to the side, making space in the centre of the pan. Add the tomatoes to the centre and cover them with the surrounding ingredients. Put the lid on and leave for 3 to 4 minutes. With the heat in the centre, and the potatoes and onion covering the tomatoes from above, they will wilt and become soft in no time.

Open the lid and stir. Add salt, cumin, and coriander powder, and mix well. Let the spices cook for one minute before adding water. Cover and cook on low heat until the potatoes are tender and cooked through. This should take about 20 to 30 minutes.

Add salt to taste and serve with coriander.

Tip: Smash some, but not all, the potatoes, to make the curry nice and thick. This makes the curry richer and creamier.

This dish is perfect with rice or *roti*. If you don't have either, you can even eat it with bread - dipping and sipping style.

8. LAUKA KO TARKARI - COURGETTE CURRY

When I've had a week of over-eating and I need a break, what I want is courgettes - Nepali-style. This is my TV meal, or my eat-in-bed-on-a-cold-day meal. Far from boring, this is comfort food, especially when eaten with rice or *roti*.

The natural sugars in courgettes makes this a very soothing and warm meal. You can cook pumpkin the exact same way.

Ingredients:

- 1 medium courgette, cubed
- 5 or 6 pieces *methi* (fenugreek seeds)
- 1 ½ teaspoon oil
- ½ teaspoon turmeric
- ½ teaspoon ginger
- Salt to taste

When the oil is hot, add the fenugreek seeds. Fenugreek seeds are usually light brown in colour, but once added to warm oil, they will begin to darken. Once the seeds are dark brown or black, add the courgette, mix and sauté for a few minutes.

Add turmeric and salt, and mix for the next few minutes. If the mixture looks like it will burn, add a dash of water. Cover and let it cook for 20 minutes, until the courgettes become soft, adding more water if necessary. Remember that courgettes will release their own water, so only add water if it looks like it might burn. Smash all of the courgettes, creating a thick consistency like mashed potatoes. Add ginger and evaporate the water, if there is any.

9. *CHAU KO TARKARI - MUSHROOM CURRY*

Curries are funny things. They follow the same rules and use similar ingredients, and you can choose to add something or to not add another. It is totally adaptable to your choice of spices, or those you have in your cupboard. The same rule of thumb applies to chicken curry as it does to mushroom curry, or curry you want to make from broccoli or sweet potato, or any other vegetable that you wish to eat.

The main thing to remember is this:

Almost all South Asian curries have garlic, ginger, onions, turmeric, and coriander, as well as both cumin powder and seeds.

Ingredients:

- 2 or 3 cups mushrooms, sliced. (I like a mix of chestnut and button mushrooms.)
- 4 medium tomatoes, finely chopped
- 1 onion, finely chopped
- 2 cloves garlic, crushed
- 1 tablespoon oil
- 1 teaspoon cumin powder
- 1 teaspoon coriander powder
- ⅓ teaspoon turmeric
- Coriander to garnish
- *Optional:* ½ teaspoon ginger, crushed

In a hot pan with oil, add ginger and garlic, and mix until the colour changes slightly. Pop in the onion and let it sweat. Do not add anything at this point, especially not salt. Salt will release the water in the onion and it won't saute as well.

Add the tomatoes, salt, turmeric, coriander, and cumin powder, cover and cook until the tomatoes are tender -

about 10 to 15 minutes. Once the mixture is nice and thick, include the mushrooms. Mushrooms don't take too long to cook, though they do release a lot of water, so make sure you dry it out. If you like it with a little bit of sauce, you can simply cook it covered for another 10 minutes.

When you turn the heat off, add some chopped coriander leaves. You can also throw in parsley, if you prefer.

Note: Mushroom curry is especially good with couscous or quinoa, or even with a side of mashed or baked potatoes. You can also jazz up your mushroom curry with some cream or coconut cream. Mushrooms pair nicely with anything creamy, so when you put the mushrooms in, add the cream. This also makes the curry sauce slightly thicker so it goes really well with the sides mentioned above.

Never boil the cream for too long though, as it will curdle on the surface of your curry, ruining the taste.

10. *KURILO KO TARKARI - ASPARAGUS CURRY*

Asparagus is not a common vegetable in the South East, but as a part of globalisation, it has become popular within the community. High in vitamins A, C and K, as well as a good source of fibre and energy, asparagus is good to have when someone is feeling slightly under the weather. While it can be grilled or sautéed with garlic and butter, what better way to enjoy asparagus than as a curry.

Asparagus curry follows the same cooking steps as the mushroom curry, and you need the exact same ingredients, so this might be a repetition for those who have already followed the mushroom curry recipe.

For those who are only interested in asparagus, here it goes again.

Ingredients:

- 2 cups asparagus, chopped
- 3 medium tomatoes, finely chopped
- 1 onion, finely chopped
- 2 cloves garlic, crushed
- 1 tablespoon oil
- 1 teaspoon cumin powder
- 1 teaspoon coriander powder
- ⅓ teaspoon turmeric
- Coriander to garnish
- *Optional:* ½ teaspoon ginger, crushed

Directions:

In a hot pan with oil, add ginger and garlic, and mix until the colour changes slightly. Next, include the onion and let it sweat. Do not put anything else in at this point, especially not salt. Salt will release the water in the onion and it won't saute as well.

Add the asparagus, salt, turmeric, coriander, and cumin powder, cover and cook until the tomatoes are tender - about 10 to 15 minutes. You want the asparagus to be cooked, but not overcooked. If you are unsure, scoop a piece of asparagus and press it against your fingers, or a fork. It should be hard enough, but not undercooked, soft but not so soft that it will fall apart when you press it against your fingers.

MEAT DISHES

My consumption of meat has really decreased since my cancer diagnosis. Nowadays, I consume mostly dairy-free and animal-free products. This is because I don't always know the quality of meat that will be served to me. Not only are animals mistreated, but they also are not raised in a good and healthy environment. They are injected with antibiotics and hormones to make them grow larger than their usual size, and forced to produce more eggs and dairy than they are supposed to.

Because of this, it was just easier for me to choose a vegetarian option, rather than having to worry about the quality of meat I was putting inside my body.

Having said that, I love to try the cuisines of different countries and cultures when I travel, and I am a Nepali after all. We love our *momos*, and meat is a very big part of our life.

During my cancer treatment, I hated the smell of meat, fish, eggs, dairy, and anything sweet. I did not eat a lot of meat, even though my mother tried to prepare some very nutritious and energy-boosting curries. In Nepali culture, it is believed that chicken soup, or *khutti ko* soup (recipe below) gives you *tagaat:* strength.

Some of you may still want to enjoy some tangy and flavourful meat curries, so here are a few Nepali recipes for you to enjoy.

Note: I would like to encourage you to try to only eat meat either from your local butcher or organic supplier. Regular meat, or "organic corn fed", is not as good. Even if it's organic, corn is not something farm animals are supposed to be eating. Sheep, goats, and cows eat grass. Chickens pick on grains and worms from the earth, while pigs feed on grains and natural protein sources. We should be eating consciously.

11. CHICKEN CURRY

Every family has their own curry recipe, and no two taste the same. This one is my particular favourite - easy to cook and full of nutrition.

Ingredients:

Serves 4

- 650g chicken
- 2 medium onions, finely chopped
- 4 to 5 medium tomatoes
- 3 tablespoons cooking oil
- 1 teaspoon garlic
- 1 teaspoon ginger
- 1 teaspoon coriander powder
- 1 teaspoon turmeric powder
- 1 teaspoon cumin powder
- ½ teaspoon *jwano (ajwain)* seeds
- ½ teaspoon cumin seed
- ¼ teaspoon black pepper
- Chilli powder to taste
- Salt to taste
- Splash of lemon

In a deep saucepan over medium heat, add cumin seeds and *jwano* seeds to hot oil. You will notice the seeds change colour and become fragrant. At this point, add the chicken and let it brown for 5 to 10 minutes.

Add turmeric and a pinch of black pepper. Mix well and add chopped onions, sauté for another few minutes until translucent. Include salt, cumin, and coriander powder, and mix well.

Make space in the middle of the pan, by moving the chicken and other ingredients to the sides of the pan. Add chopped tomatoes and chilli powder to the centre and cover it with the chicken. Pop in a cup of water, and turn the heat to low. Cover and cook for 20 to 30 minutes.

Open and check the consistency of the curry. If you want to make it thicker, cook it for another 5 of 10 minutes with the lid off. To make it thinner, throw in some water and let it cook for another 5 minutes.

Taste, and add salt if required. Squeeze some lemon on top when it is almost time to turn the heat off.

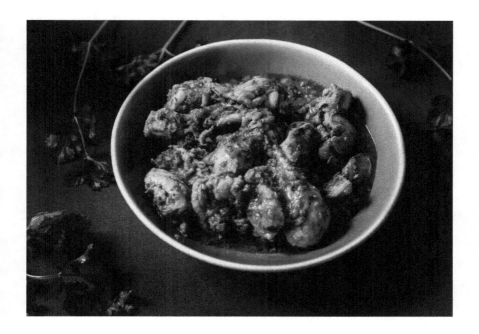

12. *KHUTTI KO JHOL - MUTTON LEG SOUP*

Mutton leg, which is mostly bone, is supposed to be full of nutrients. Make sure you ask your butcher to clean and chop it into small pieces, as it is quite difficult to do it at home.

Although to some, the sight of a mutton leg may be frightful, the taste will melt away your fears and you will want to make this as often as you can.

For mutton curries, I often used lamb meat, which is easy to find, but I am not sure if this substitute is suitable for this soup. It is not very difficult to find mutton these days. Speak to your local butcher, they might not have it all the time, but seasonally it will be available.

Ingredients:

- 2 legs of lamb/mutton or goat meat, cut into small pieces
- 2 medium onions, chopped
- 2 medium tomatoes, chopped
- 2 tablespoons mustard oil. Mustard oil is preferred, but any vegetable oil will work
- 2 bay leaves
- 1 teaspoon ginger and garlic paste, or crushed ginger and garlic
- 1 teaspoon *garam masala*
- ½ teaspoon fenugreek seeds
- ½ teaspoon turmeric
- Cumin powder, if not included in *garam masala*
- Chilli powder to taste
- Salt to taste
- Fresh coriander

This recipe is best if made in a pressure cooker, but can be done in a regular pot.

Heat some oil, and add the fenugreek seeds. Once the seeds turn dark brown, add onions and fry until browned and soft. Add the bay leaf, and mix until they become slightly soft and change shape. Add turmeric and mix well.

Add the mutton leg and mix before letting fry for about 10 minutes. Add ginger and garlic paste, salt, chilli powder, cumin and mix for a few minutes. Add tomatoes, and stir for a few more minutes. Add *garam masala* or meat *masala*.

Add water to make it soupy, with a little extra water because it needs to simmer for a long time - longer than any regular meat.

If you have a pressure cooker, cook for about 14 to 15 whistles. If using a deep-dish pan, cook for about an hour, to an hour and 20 minutes, on low heat, covered. You will know it's ready when the meat around the leg falls off the bones. When serving, sprinkle coriander on top.

13. *EGG CURRY*

Egg curry reminds me of my boarding school. As boarding school kids, deprived of good food, Wednesday was a joyous moment - because we would have egg curry for dinner.

If I were to go back and taste it now, it would probably taste inedible. It looked like they just added boiled eggs to red soup. Instead of a thick gravy, it was a thin stew, and it was easy to spot the eggs. We were only allowed two eggs per person - no more, no less.

I used to smash the yolk of the egg and mix it in with the curry, so it would be nice and thick. Then, I would cut the white of the egg into proper cubes so I could use the *roti* to dip and grab. That first bite was always surprising, because of how delicious it was.

Now, every time I eat egg curry, it reminds me of those times as a child, how happy and grateful we were for Wednesday dinners and the joy it brought when I took the first bite. It is a constant reminder that we should find joy and happiness in every small thing we can, just like a child.

Ingredients:

- 6 to 8 eggs, boiled and shelled
- 3 medium tomatoes, finely chopped
- 2 tablespoons oil
- 1 onion
- 1 teaspoon garlic
- 1 teaspoon ginger
- 1 teaspoon cumin powder
- 1 teaspoon coriander powder
- ½ teaspoon cumin seeds
- ½ teaspoon *garam masala*
- 1 teaspoon turmeric
- Salt to taste
- Pinch of *hing*

In a pan, warm one cup of oil. Once hot, add the whole boiled and shelled eggs. At this moment be very careful, as some oil might splash as the egg browns on the outside. Because of their shape, the eggs will brown unevenly, but that's okay. I also often like to fry the egg cut in half, length wise. The crispy outside gives it a great flavour later when added to the curry. Once brown on the outside, put the eggs aside.

To the same pan, temper with cumin seed and a pinch of *hing*. Blend the onion, garlic and ginger to fine paste. Add it to the pan, sauté until they are brown a bit. While you are doing this, add the tomatoes (roughly chopped) to a blender, to make a smooth paste. The thickness of the paste doesn't matter, as the consistency can be adjusted later.

Add turmeric, coriander, and cumin powder to the onion, garlic and ginger paste. Let this cook for another few minutes, until fragrant. Add the blended tomatoes to the pan and cook this for about 10 minutes.

You will see the colour of the tomato puree change, or a little bit of oil float to the surface. This means the curry is cooked. Add the eggs, and then the *garam masala*.

Add the fried eggs, simmer for another 5 minutes so the flavours are absorbed by the eggs. You can adjust the consistency of the curry at any time.

Enjoy on its own or with rice, *roti* or *naan*.

CONDIMENTS AND SALADS

14. *GOLBEDA KO ACHAAR* - *TOMATO ACHAAR*

This is the grandmother of all salsas - a condiment we eat with almost all our meals. Sometimes cooked, sometimes just grilled to soften the tomatoes, and sometimes raw.

This is what makes *momo* taste delicious, and what gives life to a whole meal. Raw, this doesn't keep for too long, but if cooked, it will last you about a week in the fridge, in a jar.

My favourite with black *daal,* or with just plain rice, this recipe will get you hooked to *golbeda ko achaar.* The natural tanginess and the combination of the well balanced salt and (natural) sugar of tomato makes it a delight with every meal, and I promise that you will end up licking the spoon (and your plate).

Every family has their own recipe for *golbeda ko acchar* and nothing is set in stone. This is one of the few things that I prefer made by my mom, even though my grandmother is usually a better cook.

Ingredients:

- 2 to 3 medium tomatoes
- 2 to 3 cloves garlic
- ½ teaspoon *timur* or *Szechuan* pepper
- 1 teaspoon lime juice
- 1 teaspoon mustard oil
- ½ teaspoon pepper
- Salt to taste
- Green or red chillies, to taste

Mustard oil is very pungent and spicy in its raw form. This gives the *achaar* its unique flavour.

If you have a gas top, grill the tomatoes and garlic over the flame. Alternatively, you can use an oven or boil a little bit of water in a pan, and add the tomatoes for a few minutes until you see the skin peeling off. Add the garlic for less than a minute before you take them off of the heat.

Either way, remove the skin. With boiled or oven-roasted tomatoes, the entire skin comes off easily. With tomatoes grilled over flames, some charred skin will remain. Do not worry - this will give your *achaar* a smoky flavour.

To put everything together, you can use a mortar and pestle or a food processor. Simply put all the ingredients together and blitz it. Remember not to make a smoothie or soup. Leave the tomatoes and garlic chunky. Taste, and add salt and lemon juice.

Note:

Do not use cherry tomatoes, kumato, or green zebra tomatoes. You can use ripe San Marzanos, better boys, roma tomatoes, beef-steak tomatoes, or even green tomatoes.

15. *AALO KO ACHAAR - POTATO ACHAAR*

This confused, yet superbly versatile dish can be a snack, a condiment, and even a meal on its own. I remember, as a child, binge eating more than I should and not being able to eat anything else. A medley of flavours, made with the world's favourite vegetable, *aalo ko achaar* goes with everything. I often make it for potlucks, and to take to friends. I have never known anyone who has not loved it.

It is also extremely simple to prepare - simply throw all the ingredients in a mixing bowl and *voila*, it's ready to be served. The only thing I often mess up is the consistency of the potatoes. They should be cooked and soft, but not so mushy that they don't hold their shape.

Aalo ko achaar is served at room temperature or cold, and it's one of those things that taste better the next day. Potatoes absorb all the goodness overnight.

Ingredients:

- ½ kg potatoes
- 4 to 5 fenugreek seeds
- ½ cucumber (optional)
- 3-4 tablespoon roasted and ground white (or brown) sesame
- 1 teaspoon turmeric
- 1 tablespoon mustard oil
- ½ to 1 teaspoon red dried chillies
- Lime
- Salt and pepper to taste
- Coriander

Boil and dice the potatoes into big cubes. Do not use potatoes that are used for mashing. The potatoes when cut should hold their shape. Place in a mixing bowl with salt, chillies, black pepper, sesame powder and cucumber - soak the cucumber in salt and squeeze the water out, so it does not make the *achaar* soggy.

In a pan, heat oil, and once the oil is hot, pop in the fenugreek seeds. You will know the seeds are done when they change colour completely. Once they are black, add red dried chillies and turmeric. Turn the heat off, and pour the mixture over the potatoes. This tempering method is used quite commonly in our cooking.

Garnish with a squeeze of lemon and a sprinkle of coriander, and mix all the ingredients well. Serve instantly or eat it the next day.

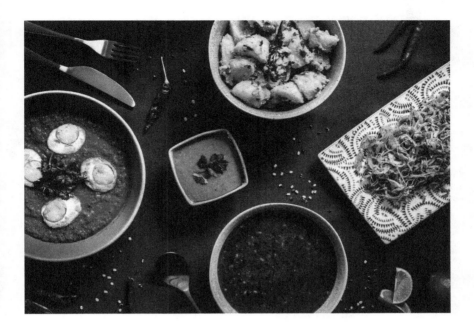

16. *Tusah (seed) salad or Sprout salad*

It is very convenient to get sprouts these days in supermarkets. Alfalfa sprouts, sky sprouts, peanut sprouts, mung bean sprouts, buckwheat sprouts - the list goes on.

Sprouts on their own can be quite strong in flavour, and you can always add them to salads or eat them the way I do, with some cucumber, tomatoes, and onions. This raw salad is not only crispy and tasty, but the freshness of the ingredients and the sourness of the lemon leaves your stomach feeling light.

Ingredients:

- 2 handfuls sprouts
- 1 small cucumber, finely chopped

- 1 large or 2 medium tomatoes, finely chopped
- 1 to 2 cloves garlic, finely chopped or smashed
- ½ onion, finely chopped
- ½ teaspoon oil (I prefer mustard oil, but you can use any you prefer)
- Lemon or lime juice to taste
- Salt and pepper to taste
- Pinch of Sichuan pepper or *timur*

Mix all the ingredients in a mixing bowl and taste. Add flavouring accordingly, and remember - this salad has to be tangy. Super easy and super appetising

You can also make this salad without the onions, tomatoes, and cucumber.

17. CABBAGE WITH IMLI

This dish is almost like a salad, though more fun and innovative. Because it is consumed cold, I'm happy to continue calling it a "salad"... Either way, it is a good way to get flavour into your food.

The sweet and sour combination of this dish is appealing to one's palate during treatment. To me especially, bland food tasted blander, and, therefore, this dish was a great condiment, or a quick bite when I wasn't hungry. It was a good way to get most of the important nutrients into my body.

Ingredients:

- 4 cups cabbage
- 4-5 tablespoons *imli*
- Sesame powder or tahini

- Black pepper to taste
- Sugar, if the *imli* is too sour
- Salt to taste
- Chillies

If you have dried *imli*, take an amount the size of your thumb and add three tablespoons of hot water. Mix and leave it for 30 minutes to form a thick liquid

Cut the cabbage into fine, long pieces. Add two heaped tablespoons of salt and mix well. Set aside and let sit for at least 30 to 45 minutes. This process takes all the water out of the cabbage so that when you add *imli*, it won't be soggy, and cabbage will remain crunchy.

Squeeze all the water out of the cabbage with your hands. The more water you can squeeze out, the better it will be.

Finally, add and mix the cabbage, sesame powder or tahini, *imli*, and black pepper in a large mixing bowl. Don't add salt yet. According to your preference, add salt, chillies, and sugar. Sometimes the *imli* can be very sour.

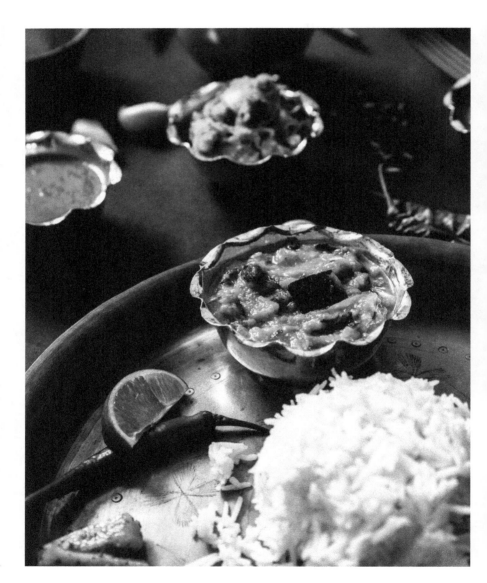

DRINKS

18. *LASSI*

A common drink in Indian restaurants, *lassi* has two functions - to calm your stomach after a spicy meal, and to and aid digestion because of the good bacteria yoghurt has. During my treatment, it aided me quite a bit. It helped to settle my stomach and the resulting gas. The chemotherapy medications, and other medications you are required to take, can do a great deal of damage to the lining of the stomach.

When I didn't feel like eating, it also served me well as a snack - a filling drink which provided the nutrition I needed.

Lassis can be either sweet or savoury.

A sweet *lassi* can be made with any fruit, mango being the most popular among my friends. Almost like a smoothie, you can add other fruits and sweet ingredients to it as well, such as bananas with cinnamon and cardamom powder, or honey and berries.

A savoury *lassi*, on the other hand, which is what I prefer, is not just made with plain salt. Rather, it can be flavoured with roasted cumin seeds and chopped fresh or dry mint. A discovery I made, and my favourite way to prepare *lassi*, is to add grated fresh or powdered *amala* (Indian gooseberries). This gives a slight bitterness and a whole lot of tanginess to your drink - also providing *amala's* immense benefits.

Sweet *lassis* are generally slightly thicker in consistency and taste better that way, while a savoury lassi is almost the consistency of juice.

19. *Chai or Chiya (and variations)*

It's difficult to say who loves tea more - the Indians or the English. It's such a fashion in the UK to drink a cuppa or more every day. Unlike their neighbours, people in the UK drink tea with milk, making it *chai* - or *chiya* as we say in Nepali.

But my friend, let me tell you, what most people drink here is not really *chai*. It is tea with a dash of milk. Let me tell you how to make a real *chai* that will blow you away.

Tea can take anywhere from 5 to 20 minutes to make, and the longer it cooks, the tastier it is. When you don't have 20 minutes to wait for a pick-me-up, here is what you can do:

Ingredients:

Makes one cup

- 1 teaspoon loose tea leaves
- 1 ½ cups water
- ½ cup milk
- Sugar, or your prefered alternative sweetener to taste

Directions:

Boil the water, and once it starts to bubble, add the tea leaves. Let it boil for another few minutes, over medium heat.

If you want to make ginger tea or *masala chai*, this is when you add spices:

- a pinch of *Mamu's garam masala*, or
- ¼ teaspoon ginger, slightly smashed, or
- 2 cardamom pods, crushed

After about 5 minutes, add milk and sugar and let it continue to boil a bit more. Make sure it doesn't spill over, which it very likely will. After the milk has risen a few times, take it off the heat, strain and sip.

Note:

It's always best to use loose tea leaves. If you like a good tasting tea, it's best to buy the ones you get in Indian stores. They are a lot darker, stronger, and make beautiful tea.

20. HOT LEMON HONEY

As the name suggests, this is just lemon and honey with hot water. It is a popular drink during the winter months, especially when one has a sore throat. You can also use lime instead of lemons, which is what we do back home, where we often refer to limes as lemons. I'm not sure when and why the name was swapped.

This drink is summer in a glass, ideal for when it's cold outside, or when you need something for your aching throat.

Ingredients:

- Juice of half a lemon
- 1 to 2 tablespoons honey
- *Optional:* ginger, chopped or roughly smashed.

Simply add the lemon juice and honey to boiling water and stir. Use raw honey if you can.

21. FRESH LEMON SODA

If hot lemon honey is for winter, lemon soda is for summer. This is not just lemon and soda water - rather, it is *Raja-fied*, making it the master of all drinks. It also helps with indigestion, or when you've had too much spicy food, and your stomach says, *"enough is enough"*.

Ingredients:

- Juice of half a lemon
- 250ml plain soda or sparkling water
- Pinch of black salt (or regular salt)

    or

- 1 tablespoon sugar syrup or honey

Lemon soda can be either savoury or sweet. If you're feeling adventurous, you can do both.

Simply combine the ingredients, and have your mind blown.

22. TAMARIND DRINK

This is a recipe shared with me by a dear Egyptian friend. Tamarind drink is very popular in Egypt and some Middle Eastern countries, as well as in the Caribbean. The traditional recipe is slightly boring, using only tamarind, sugar and water. This is a better, and slightly more fun version.

Ingredients:

- 2 tablespoons tamarind paste
- 1 teaspoon rose water
- Dash of lemon juice

- Your choice of sweetener (honey, agave, and coconut nectar are popular)

If you don't have tamarind paste, you can soak tamarind pulp in water to make your own.

Simply combine the ingredients in a glass, or place everything in a blender with water and ice for a crushed tamarind frappé.

ME

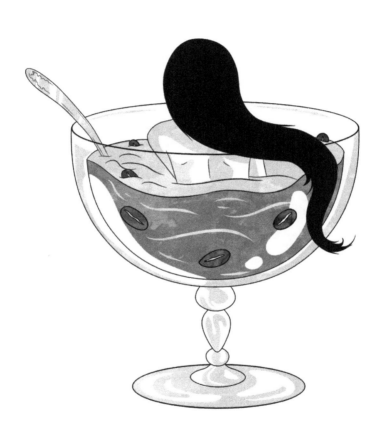

Conclusion - *Sikarni*

After the Battle

"Sikarni"- My favourite Nepali dessert, made with hung yoghurt, cream, nuts, and spices. This dessert brings together everything delicious, with spices such as nutmeg, cinnamon, clove, and cardamom. Like any dessert, sikarni concludes a meal, leaving a great taste in your mouth.

Although the struggle and recovery feel like a long process, and it can be, it all eventually comes to an end. The regular doctors' visits became less frequent, the side effects started to fade, and I began to feel okay again. Finally.

I began to look and feel a lot like my old self. But there was still this part of me that had had this extraordinary experience. I couldn't possibly go back to being my old self. Every time I looked in the mirror naked, I was haunted by my past. My wardrobe was not the only thing I had to change over this time. I had to change my outlook on life.

How did I do that? How could I suddenly change my whole philosophy?

By realising and internalising the *new* me.

For hours, days, and months on end, I reflected on what cancer had taught me. What did I learn? What am I destined to do now? How am I going to change the world...How am I going to save the world?

It seems that everyone who has gone through cancer has found a spiritual path, or had some sense of enlightenment about life's deeper meaning. Mine was still missing.

I was not a smoker. I didn't abuse alcohol. I didn't eat unhealthily. I was not lazy. There was no 'ah-ha' moment after cancer that would make me transform my life.

Studies have shown that those who smoke and are overweight are at a higher risk of cancer. But, I was in the prime of my life. I had, less than a year before, done an overall health check and all my systems seemed to function fine. So, I was certainly not "saved" by my cancer experience. It might happen to some, but for me, it didn't.

I had come to terms with the fact that me having cancer- going through this journey - might not have a bigger purpose. It just happened. And just like that, once everything begins to fall back to place, life goes on as it used to.

Once my treatments ended, I began to get back to my 'normal' life. I wanted to go back to the gym, or go travelling, or just be able to do the things I used to do before cancer. Something as simple as walking 1 km without taking a break. I wanted my hair to grow long - fast! I wanted to be able to go to yoga class and do a perfect headstand. Unfortunately, this also didn't happen.

It took me four to five months after completing my radiotherapy just to be able to regain some strength. Three years after my treatment, I still can't do a headstand. The surgery affected my nerves and I have no sensation on some parts of my breast. The internal scars and the lack of breast muscles mean I can't lift heavy things and my right arm often seems to be in pain. There are some permanent side effects of radiotherapy, which means I can never have direct sun exposure to that area of the chest. I have to be extra cautious when I go to the beach, or even with the clothes I wear in summer. But, life goes on.

I was impatient, impractical. I wanted to push myself and, in the process, I realised I was only getting weaker inside by beating myself up so much. The person who was so level-headed, thought so clearly, took rational steps during the treatment process, she had become someone else entirely.

Once everything was over, I was lost. I was doing very little work from home, which meant my mind had ample time to wander. It certainly didn't wander in the right direction. I was overweight and my body looked and felt different. Physically, I was not the same as I used to be. The people around me were constantly asking me what's next in life and when I would be working full time, or moving on. Everything hit me all at once. I was depressed.

A year of full recovery later and I knew I had to do something about it. I found a course that was offered by the Breast Cancer and Macmillan Center at the UCLH called 'Moving Forward'. That helped me more than any counselling sessions I've ever gone to. I realised that I was not alone. There were many others, two or three years after recovering, still facing the hard reality of what they went through.

Accepting and healing go hand-in-hand, for me. Healing is not only physical. It's also psychological. Not all women who have breast cancer have a mastectomy but if they do, it means dealing with body image issues and self-esteem. This also applies to those who, in some way or another, have gone through physical changes from the treatment, like side effects from chemotherapy or various medications.

Over time, my appetite improved and food actually tasted great again! My eyesight and memory seemed to get better, and binge-watching Netflix or reading a book weren't so difficult anymore. From sleeping all day to taking fewer naps - a more active routine seemed to agree with my body. Things started to fall back into place.

During this process, I began to take note of how I healed, uncovering how beautiful our bodies really are. The way they repair themselves is remarkable. I understand now how they can be affected if we don't take good care of them, or if we have to control them with pharmaceutical drugs. Those drugs saved my life, but also made me weak, ill, and almost killed me - twice in my case.

My natural physiology took over. My body re-adapted, my follicles grew new hair, my eyelashes towered long to protect my eyes, my nails grew back to shield my fingers. Never had I been happier to see hair all over my body! And nothing was better than the feeling of a pencil in between my fingers. My nails were growing and holding a pencil was not painful anymore. I could write.

Cancer was my enemy, or at least I thought it was. I cursed cancer! Hated even hearing the term, or seeing any movie where, if someone was unwell and dying, cancer was the culprit. As I came to terms with my new self, I realised that cancer was a part of me. It was a part of my body trying to teach me something.

FOOD

As a young child, I remember playing outside in my grandparents' garden, when *Pokemon Go* wasn't the only reason to be outdoors. I distinctly recall the times playing hide and seek, crouching behind a tree with a massive beehive attached to it, which obviously led to me being stung by a few honeybees. Now, in a South Asian family, your parents won't give you ibuprofen and a hug for bee stings. They'll typically make a paste with turmeric and mustard oil and apply it to your wounds - this only after a good round of yelling and being told off, of course. Surprisingly, the pain would vanish and the stung area healed in no time.

Most kids raised on the Indian subcontinent would remember someone (generally) older advising them on how spices not only taste good in their food but can also get rid of bad smells in their closet. Or, they can be used to treat pain. *Timur* or Sichuan pepper is used widely in China and Nepal to keep termites and fungus away. These are spicy life hacks we grow to love.

From my upbringing, and my journey, I have a greater appreciation for food, where it comes from, and what it does to our bodies. I have realised that what Mother Earth has offered us must not be taken for granted. In a world of quick and processed foods, I take the time to cook and eat clean. I have seen and felt the change in my body with eating a more plant-based, whole food diet, and I share that enthusiastically with people.

I have gone back to my roots - my grandmother's recipes, which are actually her grandmother's. My aunt's cooking tips and references to Ayurvedic roots has now become something that is engraved inside me.

If we talk about taking care of ourselves, we must talk about the impact food has on our bodies. I decided to give up meat, dairy, processed food, and alcohol. There are occasions where I make exceptions; like birthdays and anniversaries. If I'm celebrating, I really don't see any harm in a proper toast.

My husband has been following my diet at home. Although he is a meat lover, he has absolutely no problem eating what I eat and supporting all the drastic changes and decisions I have made. Regardless of my personal dietary choices, I do feel that everyone should try and commit to eating seasonal, local produce and to use cooking methods that do not destroy the essential components of the ingredients.

There is a growing trend in South Asia for olive oil, mostly because of its nutritional benefits and value. Nonetheless, it is not local to the South Asian region. It is not produced there and all the olive oils that are imported are not of the highest quality. In these instances, it is better to stick to what is local to the market.

In Nepali cooking, some things need to be cooked in mustard oil, some in sunflower, and some in ghee. Most of the foods cooked at higher temperatures use mustard oil and ghee because of their heat resistance, while others, like sesame oil, are used for drizzling.

Easy meals have become equated with processed food. This doesn't have to be the case. It might be tempting to make a spam sandwich rather than prepping and cooking a meal. But, if you plan and do meal preparations, making that gloopy sandwich might be just as time-consuming. We see the importance of a balanced diet everywhere. No matter what a popular diet may say, I think carbohydrates are equally as important as fats, proteins, and vitamins.

This is where traditional cooking teaches us so much. For instance, look at your typical English roast dinner. It has meat, vegetables, and potatoes, or some other form of carbohydrate. An Indian or a Nepali Thali will typically have not just the four basic tastes (sweet, salty, sour, and bitter), but six. According to Ayurveda, there are six tastes, which also include pungent and astringent. The heat of the spices, like that of ginger, mustard, or even chillies are what make a dish pungent. And the use of some ingredients, such as unripe bananas, Indian gooseberries (*amala* in Nepali, *amla* in Hindi), or okra are the astringents.

Every culture has its own age-old remedies - just ask your parents and grandparents. My English friends recommended a sachet of dry lavender by my pillow to help sleep better, or an apple as a natural toothbrush to keep stains away. My Italian friends tell me that they use fresh olive oil for practically everything, not just cooking.

Food has the ability to be a remedy, to cheer you up, and to provide what's essential to your body. We must let food heal us. The best way to do that is to go back to our roots, when processed food was not available. We need to go back to a time when we ate seasonal food grown in our backyard or from regular local vendors. We can learn so much from our ancestors and the way they ate.

We just have to listen to the old wives' tales.

LIFE

As it happens, we all have our share of grief that shapes us into who we are. Before cancer, the death of my maternal grandfather was one of my biggest life-defining losses.

In 2008, I had moved to the UK to complete my master's degree. A few weeks after the move, my maternal grandfather passed away. It was very sudden and unexpected. He was healthy, still riding his bicycle across busy Kathmandu, and gardening and farming to keep himself fit. It came as a shock to all of us, especially because I had sent him an email two days prior and received his reply within a few hours.

Dilli Raj Uprety, my *Mambaba*, was a man way ahead of his time. He encouraged his wife to work while they lived in France and in Nepal, which, in the 1960s, was unheard of. All of his grandchildren could have political, religious, and life discussions with him. Even if we had a difference of opinion, he was always proud of us.

I was unable to see him off and attend the cremation. Because of that, I never came to accept that he was gone. My heart and mind could not align and I was not able to deal with his passing. So, I had to do the one thing South Asian culture looks down on: I had to seek professional help. I had to go to therapy.

Many South Asians will understand the last statement because we believe that we do not, in any way, require therapy or psychological help. Only those with serious mental illness, where one's actions are not within one's control, will require professional mental treatment. The rest of us have friends and family.

After many sessions with the university counsellor, I began to grieve. Over time, the loss of my grandfather became my motivation and strength. I needed to continue to make him proud. Unfortunately, the process took a little longer than expected. I graduated with an unsatisfactory grade and a Master of Arts degree.

With the goal of making my grandfather proud and continuing his legacy, I decided to go back to university. But this time, I would only attend one of the top universities in the world. It was this same fire in me that led me to make my life after cancer meaningful.

Mambaba always thought I was a great storyteller. When I decided to write, all I could think of was him telling me that I would be a great writer someday. Within the perils of self-doubt and the desire to raise awareness, I started this book.

With or without *Mambaba*, life moved on. It was my determination to keep positive memories of him alive that kept me motivated and helped me appreciate him even more. It is this same positive thinking that I saw transform my life during treatment.

I decided to choose the path of 'life is great no matter what'. It wasn't always. I had to train my mind to see the good in almost everything. At first, it was impossible, then it became difficult, later it came naturally. Not only did training my mind to think positively help me, my family, and others around me have a different experience with cancer, but I noticed that my physical health improved.

Do you believe in the power of the mind?

I have become a firm believer after my cancer experience. Let me give you an example which is not mine. My dear mother is a clean freak. She is very particular about hygiene, cleanliness, tidiness, and is certainly quite overwhelming to those who get to know her for the first time.

Her nose twitches and her smile becomes crooked when she doesn't approve of someone's hygiene practices, although she might not say anything. This is particularly a problem when we go for dinners and eat outside. My mother is the person who always inspects glasses, plates, and cutlery for any marks or grime. She is under the impression that she always gets dirty utensils. And guess what? She always does. It is actually now a joke and not even a surprise anymore. She is unhappy, complains, and frequently talks about how it's always her. And it always is. It's like her mind is asking for it.

If someone thinks they are always unhappy, unfortunate events occur and that makes them unhappy. It's like the universe is listening.

So much research has been done on the matter. Information is available all over the Internet. Many books have been written about this kind of manifestation. Regardless of what research has been done and what people say about it, I came to know firsthand the capacity for our brains to make things happen.

Positive thinking is not only about being happy, upbeat, and energetic all the time. It creates real value and manifests in our lives with substantial impact.

My recovery was something that even the medical team was surprised by. Very few people, apparently, make quick progress and recover the way I did.

Every day, I sat for about 20 minutes and listed all the things I was grateful for. I preferred doing this before bed because I noticed that I woke up satisfied and somewhat happier the next day. I chose to only speak with my friends who were positive and optimistic, and for some time, I avoided any conversation that would lead the other way. I read books and watched TV shows that made me laugh, rather than the psychological thrillers that I generally love.

I kept asking myself what I want and how I can get there. From wanting something small, to bigger goals in life. My future. One of my goals during my treatment was to be able to walk two blocks instead of one, because walking one block was challenging. When I achieved that, I rejoiced. I was over the moon! I was so happy that the effect of my happiness also impacted my husband and parents who were taking care of me. I refused to let myself think for a second that, six months previously, walking five miles was easier than the two blocks I just did. The triumph was still mine.

I tried to keep my mind away from the negative and focused on the positive. This eventually manifested in my actions, my physical health, and everything around me becoming balanced and good.

I was one of those people who often believed that, when one thing goes wrong, everything else collapses.

I proved myself wrong this time. Training my mind made positive thoughts propagate and I think everyone around me could see and feel that difference.

The most amazing personal example I can give you is really a small miracle to me. Last year, Raj and I were going to try and start a family. I had to stop my endocrine therapy and let my body get rid of the toxins. Six months after I stopped my medicines, I went to see a gynaecologist. She examined me and said that my ovaries were 'asleep' and might never wake up but that there are always exceptions. This meant that my ovaries were not going to work or be able to produce eggs. This was because of chemotherapy.

We accepted the fact that we might not be able to conceive naturally, so decided to opt for Invitro Fertilisation (IVF). In October 2019, when I was supposed to go to initiate the process of IVF, they did a blood test and said I was pregnant. To our surprise - and the doctors' - they decided to do a scan to confirm the results. I was pregnant but unfortunately it was an ectopic pregnancy. It was quite serious and I was rushed into surgery to remove my right fallopian tube (salpingectomy) and the embryo that had settled in the tube.

A few months later, when we were ready to begin IVF again, I was pregnant again! This time, it was a normal pregnancy. Now as I complete the last few pages of my book, we await the birth of our daughter in September 2020. Both of these unexpected pregnancies were natural.

I think this story gives hope. It tells me that a body can heal and a mind can facilitate that healing process. My husband and I were not hung up on the fact that I might never conceive again, but rather looked forward to options that were available to us. Although the ectopic pregnancy wasn't a pleasant add-on after what I had overcome not too long ago, it was a reminder that this is life. We face numerous hurdles and we just have to overcome them.

Awareness

Can I admit one of my biggest embarrassments? I did not know what breasts or breast cancer were called in Nepali, until I was diagnosed with the illness and I asked my dad. Although it's my mother tongue and I speak it fluently, growing up we spoke colloquial Nepali- which includes a lot of slang, informal words, and a whole lot of English. But, that is not the only reason that I didn't know what a breast was called in Nepali.

It is also because, as a society, talking about breasts is not common - it is taboo. My mother or grandmother were the only people who would tell me what they were called. Even they referred to breasts as *'chati'*, which literally translates to 'chest' in English. Talking about reproductive organs in our culture is frowned upon. Even among women, it is discouraged and socially awkward to discuss it. Someone who speaks openly about reproductive organs is either a doctor or a pervert. It was only once I had breast cancer that I asked my father what it was called in Nepali, and of course, very hesitantly, he told me 'stan'.

When I wrote my first article that was published in Nepal's leading English newspaper, it was titled 'Let's Talk About Breasts'. My father and mother discouraged me from using the word 'breasts' because they were worried about how it would be received by readers. I wanted to shock my readers, and by eliminating the term, it would have lost its impact. And I was right. I think it was well received.

Since my cancer journey, one of the reasons I talk about cancer, write articles, and try to help others is because I believe awareness is important. I had no visible side effects but I was able to detect cancer at an early stage because when I looked at my breast in the mirror, it looked different.

Most women in South Asia are so ashamed of their bodies that looking at them is not something that is done regularly. The taboo around reproductive health, which also includes the breasts, is a problem. Studies even show that women or girls who are body-shamed or not happy with their own bodies, have a higher chance of getting cancer because they do not look at themselves enough, if at all.

Parents don't speak to their children about it and it certainly is not a part of the syllabus in schools. With cancer on the rise, I hear cases of younger people being diagnosed. It is important to know about cancer. If you detect it early enough, you can save lives.

Girls need to be aware of the early signs and symptoms of breast cancer. After they get their periods, they should be taught to do a regular self-examination of their breasts. Feel them, cup them, caress them, and make sure to know how they feel and look generally. If they don't look the same, they'll know when to ask for help. Not every change to our body is cancer, but knowing when something is different is important.

Cancer is treatable if detected early. Chances of survival are a lot higher than they were even 10 years ago. There is a need to know more about cancer, hear more positive stories, and know that the world of medical science is constantly changing.

I do not believe that 'everything that happens, happens for good' but I do believe that everything that happens teaches us something. It is up to us to take it as good or bad and apply it to our lives. My right foob is a constant reminder of the greatness of life, the power of my mind, the capacity of resilience, and the beauty of healing. It is also a reminder that I am loved, and of the capacity I have to love others and things around me. To appreciate life and to actually live.

"The wound is the place where the light enters you"- Rumi.

My cancer is that wound.

ABOUT THE AUTHOR

Suvekchya Ghimire was diagnosed with cancer in 2016 when she was 32 years young. Her life-altering diagnosis occurred while she was in the midst of completing her postgraduate degree at the University of Oxford. She was also working for a prestigious charity at the time.

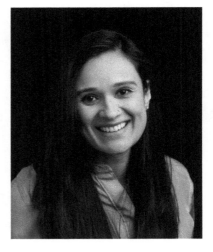

After making a full recovery, Suvekchya was able to claim back her life and graduate. She now dedicates her life to raising awareness and speaking about breast cancer, with the goal of eliminating cultural taboos surrounding the topic. She is especially drawn to a younger audience; those who may be looking for a more honest experience-share to connect with. She writes articles in both Nepali and English, speaks at events, and is available for one-to-one sessions.

Suvekchya was born and raised in Nepal and currently lives in London with her husband.

CPSIA information can be obtained
at www.ICGtesting.com
Printed in the USA
LVHW081001211020
669187LV00033B/4